sit to get fit

For Charlotte, Teddy and Dave, thanks for keeping me on my toes!

And for all my wonderful personal training clients and yoga students, who proved to me that movement is medicine and good posture is truly transformative.

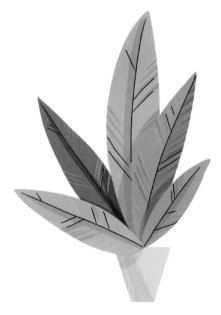

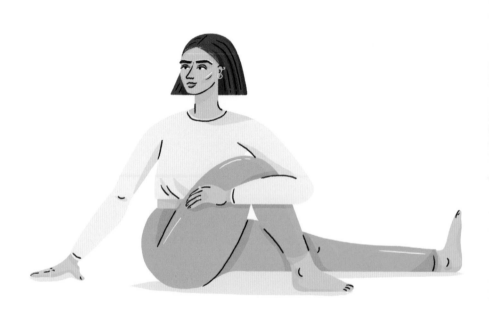

sit to get fit

Change the way you sit in 28 days
for health, energy and longevity

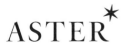

Suzy Reading

First published in Great Britain in
2022 by Aster,
an imprint of
Octopus Publishing Group Ltd
Carmelite House
50 Victoria Embankment
London EC4Y 0DZ
www.octopusbooks.co.uk

An Hachette UK Company
www.hachette.co.uk

Distributed in the US by
Hachette Book Group
1290 Avenue of the Americas
4th and 5th Floors
New York, NY 10104

Distributed in Canada by
Canadian Manda Group
664 Annette St.
Toronto, Ontario, Canada M6S 2C8

ISBN 978-1-78325-445-3

A CIP catalogue record for this book
is available from the British Library.

Printed and bound in China

10 9 8 7 6 5 4 3 2 1

Consultant publisher: Kate Adams

Senior editor: Pauline Bache

Copyeditor: Jane Birch

Art director: Yasia Williams-Leedham

Illustrator: Abi Read

Assistant production managers:
Lucy Carter and Nic Jones

Contents

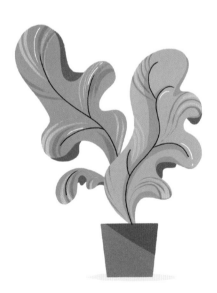

Introduction

We all know we need to move our bodies to feel fit and healthy: 70 years of comprehensive research into the benefits of movement means we've got that message loud and clear. But exercise is just one part of the solution to feeling good. Living through lockdown in 2020–21 may well have alerted you to the damaging effects of sedentary life and how we sit – whether that's at our desks, scrolling on our phones, in the car or even on our bicycles.

The average person in the UK sits for 9.5 hours a day – and in the US it's closer to 10 hours – and spends just 2 hours a week being physically active. That's only 2 hours of activity compared with 70 hours of sitting. These days, we sit on average for 3 hours more each day than we did just 20 years ago.

It's not just the recent radical changes to how we live our lives that have cultivated this more sedentary lifestyle. The trend towards sitting for big chunks of our day has been apparent for decades, and has only been amplified by the restrictions of the global pandemic.

Advances in technology have literally revolutionized how we move through our day. It may have begun with the humble television remote control, but it has now evolved into sophisticated voice-activated gadgets, allowing us to modify our environment without even lifting a finger. Strolling the malls and supermarket aisles has been

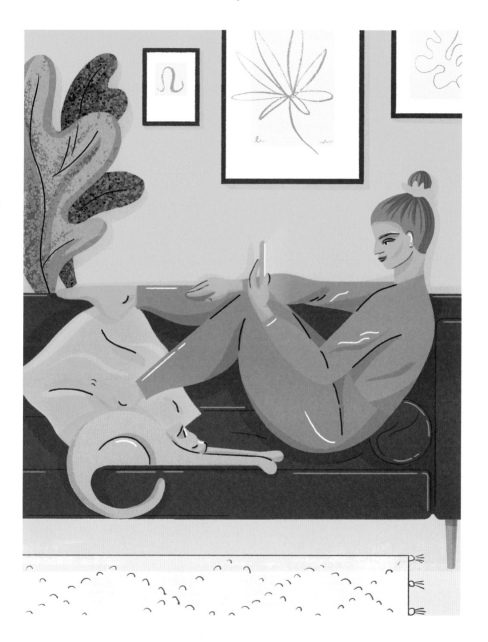

replaced by scrolling online, purchasing with the click of a mouse button from the comfort of your sofa. The advent of video calls and social media communities gives us the option to connect with others without ever leaving home.

Laptops, smart phones, email and WhatsApp groups make the "9–5" a genuine relic of the past. Our working day has been transformed: we are switched on and plugged in around the clock, which silently zaps our energy and eats into precious time for other pursuits, such as movement.

Where we work, how we work and the very nature and rhythms of our day have changed beyond all recognition over the last few decades. There are long commutes for office workers, who are then deskbound all day… and that's if we leave the house at all. According to the American Heart Association, since 1950, sedentary jobs have increased by 83 per cent. In 1960 about half the US workforce was physically active, now that figure is less than 20 per cent[1].

It's not just our work life that poses a threat to our health; according to Ofcom, the UK's broadcasting regulatory body, the average UK adult watches almost 30 hours of TV per week[2]. Downtime has become synonymous with sedentary screen time, and culturally we are constantly invited to "please take a seat". Technology and lifestyle may have evolved at lightning speed, but we're all housed in bodies perfectly designed for hunter-gatherer life. Our own physical evolution just can't keep pace.

In all the chaos of recent years, you may have seen the message broadcast over social media: "other generations have been called to war, we have been called to stay at home and sit on the sofa"[3]. However, being anchored to the sofa has its own unique and very real challenges to our well-being. Incidental movement has gone out of the window, reduced to trips to the kitchen or the bathroom. Worldwide, within 10 days of a nation's pandemic lockdown, there was a 5.5 per cent decrease in average daily steps, and within 30 days, a 27.3 per cent decrease[4].

The chorus of voices emerging from lockdown reported feeling more sluggish, rotund, achey, creaky, tight, tense and jittery than ever before. And it's crucial to note that even those who met guidelines for daily healthy movement were not immune to the creeping perils of too much sitting.

This is what the research is showing us, but the whole picture is more nuanced. The full spectrum of analysis – from examining the active sitting posture of tribesmen to the biofeedback research on the effects of "tech posture" – shows us it's not just the sedentary life that's bad for us, it's *how* you sit that matters too.

Studies into the consequences of too much sitting have led the media to claim – for good reason – that "sitting is the new smoking". We've learned first-hand through lockdown that a sedentary lifestyle is a sure-fire recipe for fatigue and muscular tension, which puts the kibosh on zest, confidence and a buoyant mood.

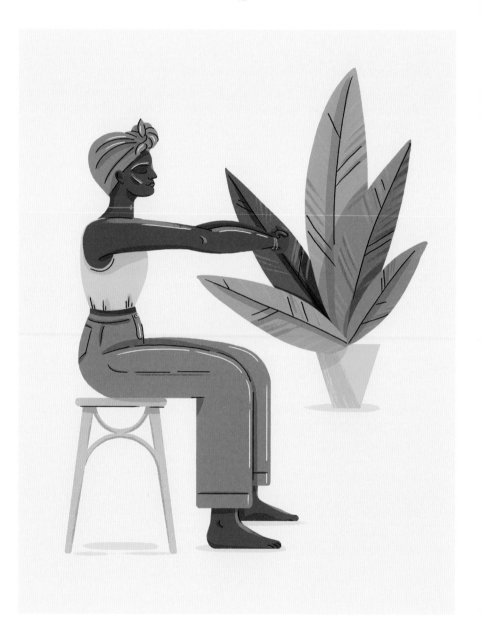

It is clear that we need to take action: we need to minimize the harm of unhealthy sitting by addressing our posture; we need practical strategies to break up sedentary periods; and we need inspiring ways to inject more movement into our daily lives once more.

As a psychologist, yoga teacher and personal trainer, I am uniquely placed to help you "sit to get fit". In this book, I'll help you to develop your mindfulness muscles – to become aware of your posture, to notice how long you've been sitting for, to create awareness of tension and stress, and to spot your body's early warning signs before they manifest as injuries or conditions that need more serious intervention. I will also help you understand the psychology behind behaviour change and show you how to form sustainable healthy habits. As a yoga teacher, I can empower you with the knowledge of healthy posture, as well as teach you how to breathe well and dial down stress. Drawing on my personal training expertise, I will share exercises to improve your posture and provide practical movement inspiration to reduce your periods of inactivity.

In this book, we will work through a concrete plan of action in 28 days that will help you to make lasting healthy changes to how you sit and move.

What have we learned?
The research round-up

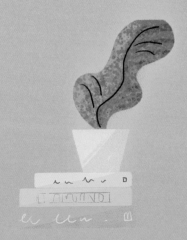

The health benefits of exercise have been clearly
demonstrated since the 1950s, with studies examining
the difference between workers who sat for prolonged
periods and those whose jobs required physical activity.
Sedentary bus drivers[5], mail sorters[6] and rail workers[7] were
shown to have a twofold greater risk of cardiovascular
disease than their more active counterparts – the bus
conductors, mail delivery workers and rail manual
workers. But it's not until more recent times that this has
been understood in context: it's not just that movement
is beneficial, it's that sedentary life is genuinely harmful.
Prolonged periods of sitting have been linked to cancer[8],
Alzheimer's disease[9], obesity, heart disease, poor
cholesterol profiles, type-2 diabetes[10] and osteoporosis[11].

In 2008, there were rumblings in the scientific community
that the issue was not just too little exercise, but also too
much sitting, with researchers stating that it was "time
to consider excessive sitting a serious health hazard"[12]
and arguing that those risks are still relevant for those
who regularly exercise[13]. In 2010, researchers began
demonstrating that small breaks in sedentary time could
have a significant impact. A higher number of breaks
is positively associated with waist circumference, body
mass index and triglyceride (a type of fat) levels[14]. (High
levels of triglycerides are associated with increased risk of
heart disease, heart attack, stroke, diabetes, obesity and
problems with the liver and pancreas.) So, in addition to
reducing time spent sitting, interrupting it helps, too.

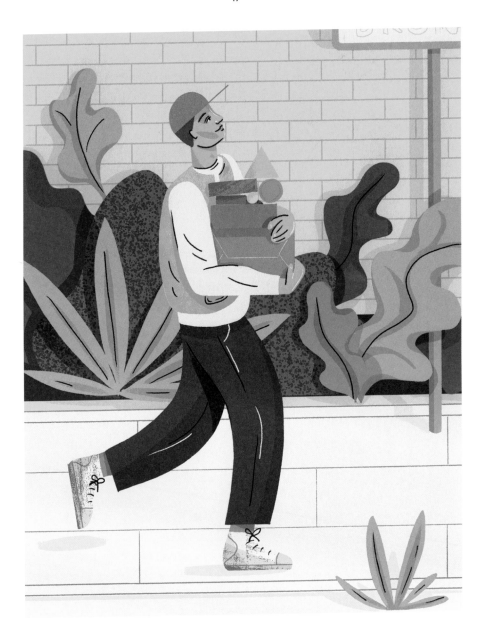

But it wasn't until 2012 that the world really stood to attention and grasped the dangers of sitting, when a team of researchers from Harvard University aimed to quantify the effect of a sedentary lifestyle on major non-communicable diseases. The landmark paper concluded that prolonged periods of inactivity killed more than 5 million people every year globally[15], a similar rate to smoking and obesity, leading to those headlines around the world claiming that "sitting is the new smoking"[16].

This was supported by another report in 2018 studying 122,000 patients, where it was found that long periods of sitting were a massive risk factor for death, more dangerous than the risk associated with smoking, diabetes or heart disease[17]. The researchers concluded that a sedentary lifestyle should be seen as a disease. A team at Queen's University Belfast and Ulster University in Northern Ireland released a sobering report in 2019[18] on the direct healthcare costs of sedentary behaviour in the UK, stating that prolonged sitting is linked to around 70,000 deaths per year, resulting in huge costs of £0.7 billion per year to the National Health Service for treating the health consequences.

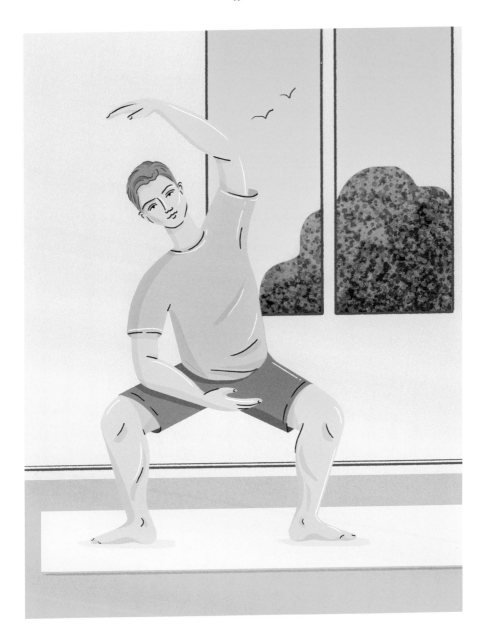

It's the way we sit

But it's not just the act of being seated, it is the way we sit in modern times that is so damaging. The advent of chairs about 5,000 years ago wreaked havoc with our bodies. When we are seated, we turn off the muscles in our legs and core, reducing the suppleness of our sinews and the range of motion in our joints, making it harder and harder to engage in the "active sitting" postures of our ancestors. Research on the hunter-gatherer Hadza community in Tanzania[19] confirms that it's not just sitting less, but how we sit that makes a difference. The Hadza had very similar patterns of movement and inactivity to Westerners, but their blood profiles and blood pressures were significantly different. While the Hadza spent nearly 10 hours a day resting, they spent 20 per cent of that rest time in "active sitting" postures, with their knees bent and their bottom off the ground, a posture that recruits leg muscles as much as 40 per cent as the act of walking. Their squatting postures meant that their bodies were not completely at rest, so they used 5–10 times more activation in their leg and core muscles than we do when taking a seat.

After a lifetime of sitting in chairs, few Westerners have the flexibility required in the feet, ankles, knees, hips and spine to engage in active sitting like the Hadza on their haunches. But we can certainly seek opportunities to stand rather than sit. We can reclaim the flexibility to sit as nature intended

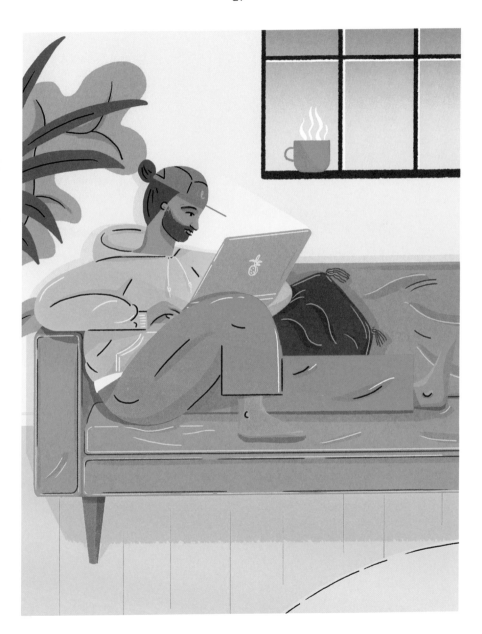

– at least for short periods – and we can break up longer stretches of sedentary time.

Recent research suggests that as little as 11 minutes of moderate- to vigorous-intensity physical activity can counter the negative effects caused by sitting, but a daily goal of 30–40 minutes leads to the most longevity gains[20]. This exercise can be taken in frequent tiny bursts spread throughout your day: astonishingly, as little as 4 seconds of high-intensity movement can reverse the damage caused by sitting[21]. And if you don't have time to hit those targets during the week, research shows that you can load all your movement into the weekend and still get the benefits[22].

It's not just physical health that's affected by inactivity and poor posture. In 2016, researchers took a group of healthy individuals in their early 20s and asked them to be more sedentary. After just 2 weeks of enforced sedentary behaviour, the group showed increased stress levels and depressive symptoms[23]. It is crystal-clear that we need to break up periods spent sitting for the sake of our mental health. The posture we adopt while sitting down makes a difference to how we feel, too. Research from psychologist Erik Peper shows that a tall upright posture boosts both mood and energy levels, whereas a rounded spine and downcast gaze (think "smart phone slump") reduce your mood and energy levels and make it easier to recall negative memories[24]. Watch Amy Cuddy's TED talk on power poses for an engaging look at the effect that posture has on your confidence, and get ready to experience it for yourself in your 28-day plan.

The health consequences of sitting in chairs

○ Sitting in chairs requires less muscle engagement, thinning our bones, weakening our muscles and reducing our muscle mass, which then has a knock-on effect of lowering metabolism and interfering with blood-sugar regulation.

○ Sitting reduces circulation, diminishing the availability of nutrients and oxygen and impeding the removal of waste products, leading to swelling, stiffness and pain in joints and muscles.

○ Sitting harms cardiovascular health by elevating triglycerides and altering the blood vessel functioning. Blood vessel walls become stiffer, making them more prone to coronary heart disease.

○ Sitting reduces our digestive health by diminishing our capacity for diaphragmatic breathing, which in turn can lead to constipation and bloating. This is because the diaphragm acts as bellows, providing a massaging action that moves waste toward the bowels.

- Inactivity leads to immune dysfunction. We need movement to help mechanically pump lymph around the body. If we don't move, the lymph doesn't move, leading to fatigue and sluggishness.

- Sitting still, coupled with slouching (as shown in the illustration on page 29), increases negative mood, stress and depressive symptoms. This could be due to the inflammation caused by immobility and its associated capacity for diaphragmatic breathing.

- Tech stress (the physical and mental strain caused by screen use) and the pressure of poor posture leads to a raft of aches, pains, tension and injuries, specifically for the spine, neck, shoulders, wrists and hands. These low levels of chronic tension disrupt quality sleep, and lead to shallow breathing, eye strain and headaches. The forward head posture created by screens reduces blood supply to the brain, leading to fatigue and stress. Equally, the diminished range of motion for the head to turn and scope the scene around us[25] potentially makes us feel subconsciously more vulnerable to threat... and anxious as a result, though we can't pinpoint the reason.

HOW CAN WE PROTECT OUR HEALTH, ENERGY AND LONGEVITY?

1. Improve posture while sitting, standing and moving.

2. Optimize our environment to support us in sitting well.

3. Break up sedentary periods with micro-moments of movement while seated, and commit to longer standing breaks that provide the antidote to sitting – strengthening our legs, core muscles and back, getting our blood pumping and enhancing our flexibility. Don't worry if you don't know where to start, you'll get plenty of fresh and achievable inspiration in your 28-day plan!

4. Undo the strain and tension caused by sitting. We achieve this with:

   • Stretching exercises

   • Breathing practices

   • Restorative practices to revive and to release stress

   • Practices to boost circulation and digestion

Posture 101

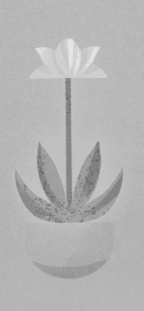

THREE STEPS TO IMPROVING YOUR POSTURE

1. Insight: awareness of how you are holding your body and knowledge of what healthy posture looks and feels like.

2. Strength: developing the muscles responsible for holding you upright.

3. Flexibility: increasing suppleness so you can sit, stand and move with more freedom.

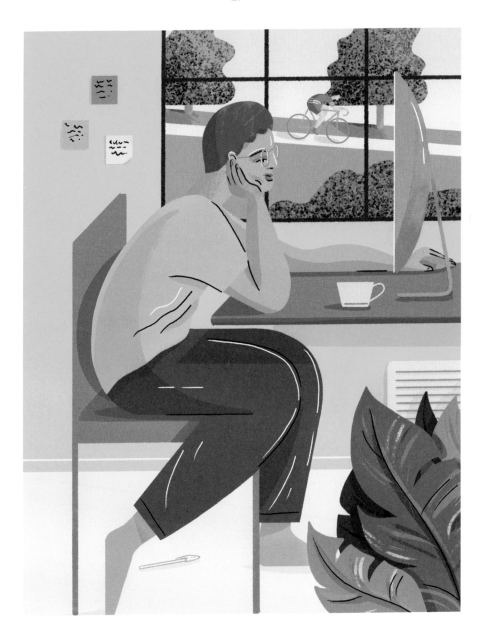

What is good posture?

Rather than explain posture in complex anatomical terms, I want to bring it to life by describing how it feels, beginning with the ideal standing position:

Starting from the ground up, place your feet hip-width apart with your toes pointing forward and your weight spread evenly between your right and left feet. Lift up all your toes, fan them out and extend them back down lightly. Your toes help you balance, rather than bearing weight. Distribute your body weight evenly between the inner and outer edges of your feet and between the balls and heels of your feet. Keep a little softness in your knees so the joint is not locked, allowing the muscles in the front of your thighs to gently hug your thigh bones.

Imagine your pelvis is a bowl – healthy posture keeps it level, so there is a feeling of containment in your lower abdomen. If your tailbone sticks out behind you, the bowl tips forward. If you tuck your tailbone under, the bowl spills backward. A subtle lift through the pit of the abdomen, created by drawing your navel toward your spine, keeps the bowl of your pelvis level. We will greet these core muscles on Day 7 of your 28-day plan (see page 72).

Feel your whole ribcage lift evenly, front and back, both sides, away from your hips. Slide your shoulder blades flat against your back, broadening your chest and bringing

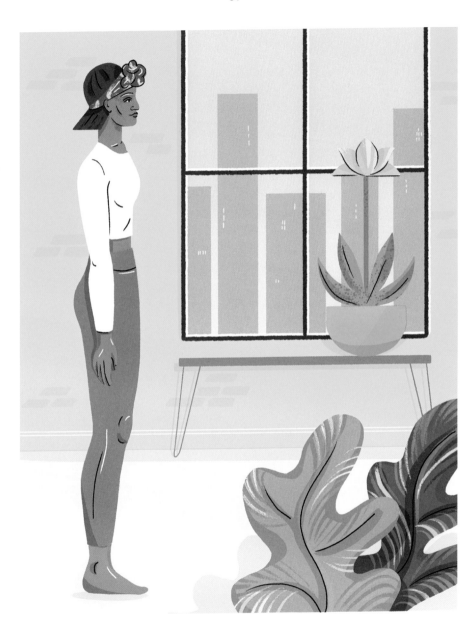

your arms to hang with your middle finger aligned with the mid-line of your outer thigh. Elongate your neck, lower your jaw parallel to the floor and snake the crown of your head skyward. Cast a soft gaze forward.

Now imagine there is a pane of glass in front of you and behind you so you can't arch your back like a soldier or round your spine in a "smart phone slump". You can only send "roots" down through your legs and feet, elevate your ribcage and blossom the crown of your head upward. Feel these equal opposites of grounding and ascension, bringing balance and symmetry to your body, lifting your mood and energy, creating freedom to breathe and space and support for the healthy functioning of your internal organs. In this "neutral spine" position, you maintain the three natural curves of the spine – at the lower back, mid-back and neck – stacking your head above your shoulders and the top of your shoulders above your hips. Your 28-day plan will develop your ability to come naturally and easily into this aligned posture.

What is healthy sitting?

For us to sit in a way that protects our health, we need to be mindful of our posture and cultivate the right environment to assist us in maintaining good spine alignment. It is important to note that even when we get the ergonomics and posture correct, we still need to break up periods of inactivity, whether that's with a few restful moments of self-massage, stretching or breathing, simply standing up, or engaging in a few minutes of dynamic movement.

The general guideline is to move every 30 minutes. Aim to factor in at least 20 and ideally 35 minutes of daily exercise to help mediate the harmful effects of inactivity. The more you break up sitting with movement the better, and, rather than hampering productivity, it will boost your focus, energy and mood.

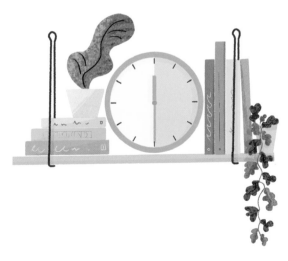

The healthiest way to sit while working

To create an environment that supports our health while sitting at screens, we need to consider the design and layout of our workspace, including the desk, chair, computer monitor, keyboard, mouse and the quality of environmental factors such as light, noise and temperature. Everyone is different, so we need to adapt our environment to suit our own specific needs and preferences.

Organize your environment to be tailored to your body – your height and proportions. You need to find a chair and desk set-up that works for you. Different types of set-up to consider include office chairs with adjustable seat height and back support, stools that encourage more activation of the core muscles, kneeling chairs, or sit/stand desks where you alternate sitting with standing to break up sedentary periods. Long periods of standing also come with health risks, so variation and mindfulness are key.

There are many different factors to consider with your set-up – the placement of the monitor and keyboard, the height and angle of your seat and its back support, as well as support for your arms. The arrangement you are aiming for allows your muscles to be held in a neutral position so you can work efficiently and reduce strain. For example, the height of arm rests can interfere with the natural alignment of your arms, causing you to tense your neck and shoulder muscles. A chair without arm rests can be better than one with arm rests at an awkward height that doesn't fit with your individual proportions.

Feeling safe is also vital for our well-being. The best-case scenario is to set yourself up so that you can easily scope the scene around you and maintain the level of privacy that you need to feel at ease. Maximize your comfort by making sure there is good access to natural light and fresh air, and try to create an optimal temperature.

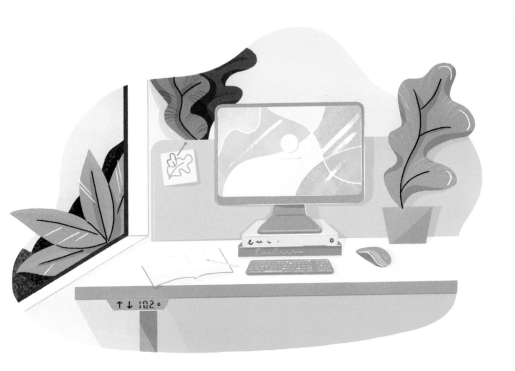

ERGONOMICS CHECK LIST

Adjust your set-up so you can:

- Place your feet flat on the floor, with a right angle at your hips and knees, using a box or footrest if necessary. Having the feet flat gives you a broad and even base of support, helping you lift up through the spine. Crossing your legs tends to make you slouch and impedes circulation. However, it is unlikely to do any long-term damage, unless you are at risk of blood clots, and in fact it can actually reduce lower back pain and sciatica by stretching the piriformis muscles (a flat band-like muscle running from your sacrum to your thigh bone). If you prefer to cross your legs, make sure you are mindful of your spine alignment. Change the cross regularly to avoid creating imbalances in strength and flexibility, and move often to avoid circulatory problems. To facilitate the right angle at your hips, you may need to adjust your seat angle so it tilts slightly downward at the front and ideally provides roughly 5cm (2 inches) space between the edge of your seat and the back of your knees. If you are using a stool, you may need to add a wedge-shaped pillow to ensure your knees are slightly lower than your hips.

- Rest your forearms on your desk so that there is a right angle at your elbow. Your forearms and wrists should be level and able to rest flat on the surface, without having to wing your elbows out or raise your shoulders up. The key is to avoid holding your wrists in a chronic flexed position, which increases the risk of carpal tunnel syndrome or tendonitis, so check the angle of your keyboard. The less you have to reach your arm to the mouse, the better.

- Sit tall, maintaining the three natural curves of the spine, with the crown of the head centred, your gaze forward and your jaw parallel with the floor. Bringing the head forward adds significant extra strain to the neck and spine, and reduces blood supply to the brain, so whether your chair has back support or not, the key is to avoid creating a "C" shape through the spine.

- Whether sitting or standing, have your monitor at eye level, the top of the screen level with your eyebrows. If using a laptop, you may benefit from adding an external keyboard and laptop stand to lift the screen to eye level. Ensure you can see print on the monitor comfortably, using the zoom function if necessary rather than squinting or craning your neck. Ideally your monitor should be an arm's length away. If you're using a smart phone or tablet, add a well-positioned holder so you're not straining your neck to look down or tensing your shoulders trying to bring the screen to eye level.

- Remember to clean the monitor to reduce eye strain. A light source coming from the side will minimize any reflection problems.

- Stretch your legs out and move your feet under your workstation. Avoid desks with drawers, as they can hamper this free movement. Some grand and elaborate chairs tend to make you feel cocooned; while they might feel super comfortable, they will limit your ability to make small adjustments and therefore actually add to the risk of impeding circulation. We don't want to feel captured by our furniture, so make sure you feel you have freedom to move in your set-up.

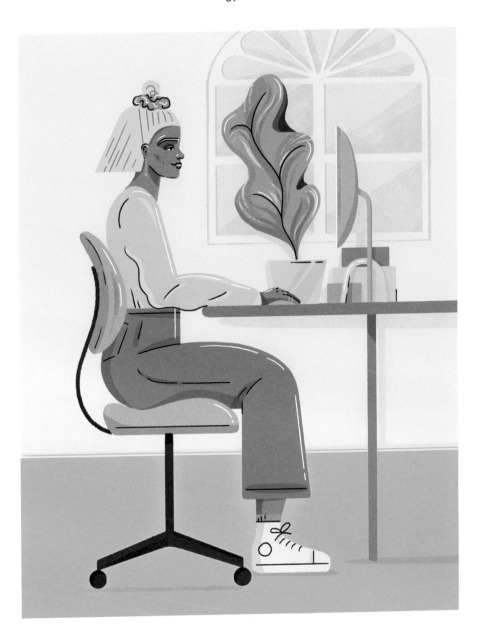

The healthiest way to sit in a car

Sitting in your car is no different from being seated at your desk, so the same guideline of ideally taking a movement break every 30 minutes applies here too, wherever practical. Stopping at a red light gives you the opportunity to check in with your body and release tension, as well as to take a couple of relaxed breaths. Just as we adapt our work environment to suit our proportions, we need to modify our driving environment, considering the vehicle's seat height and position, back and head support, steering wheel and wing-mirror location.

Run through this check list to optimize posture while driving:

- **Seat height and position:** check that your hips are at least as high as your knees and ensure that you have clear vision of the road and driving instruments, with comfortable clearance for your head. Use a wedge cushion if the maximum seat height isn't sufficient. Make sure that you can easily reach the pedals without needing to move your back away from the seat, while maintaining a small bend in your knees when the pedals are fully depressed. Make sure your thighs are supported while allowing a two–three-finger gap between the back of your knees and the front of your seat.

- **Back support:** check the angle of your seat back: a slight tilt is all that's needed. Leaning back too far will force you to push your head and neck forward and increase the pressure on your lower back. If there is adjustable lumbar support, make sure it is positioned in the small of your lower back, filling the gap, or, if your seat doesn't provide support, consider investing in a lumbar cushion. When turning the steering wheel, you should be able to keep your shoulders in contact with the seat rather than hunching them forward.

- **Head support:** adjust the head rest so it is at the same height as the top of your head. It should touch the back of your head when you're sitting comfortably in "neutral" position, to help protect you from potential whiplash injuries in the case of a collision.

- **Steering wheel:** check you can comfortably reach your wheel and that its position allows a clear view of the dashboard. Use a light grip on the steering wheel, keeping both hands on it to reduce imbalance in muscle engagement, and make sure you have a gentle bend in your elbows. Holding your hands at the clock face of "9 and 3" affords you the ideal leverage on the steering wheel, but if this creates tension in your neck and shoulders, you could try holding the wheel lower down at "7 and 4".

- **Rear-view and wing mirrors:** adjust your mirrors so you have optimal rear visibility behind you without having to crane your neck

- **Seat belt:** adjust the height to ensure your lap belt is secure over the pelvic region, not the abdomen, and the diagonal strap is hugging the clavicle and sternum, never your neck.

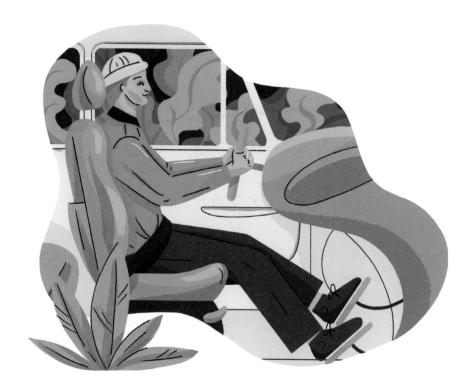

The healthiest way to sit on a bike

No adjustment can fix a bike that's the wrong size for you, so make sure your bike frame is the correct size for your proportions. Position your seat so that your knee is just slightly bent when the pedal is in its lowest position. While you don't want to strain to reach the pedals, too much knee bend is tougher on the joints and results in less efficiency. The seat itself should be level or, at most, angled a few degrees forward, never tipped backward.

You should be able to reach your handlebars and brakes comfortably with a slight bend in your elbow, reducing shoulder strain and helping you ride with less pressure in your hands. Keep your shoulders relaxed and away from your ears, allowing you to move your head freely and stay alert. While we need a bend in the elbow for shock absorption, we don't want a bend in the wrist. Aim for a straight line from your elbow through to your fingers to keep circulation flowing and stability in the joints. Make sure you keep your spine in neutral, core muscles engaged, throughout your ride.

Riding a bike might be hard work, but it shouldn't be uncomfortable. Pain, numbing or tingles, especially in the hands, feet or bottom, are a sign either that your bike set-up needs tweaking, or that you need to fire up your core muscles for greater stability and support.

The healthiest ways to sit on the floor

While we know that active squatting (see page 20) is good for muscle activation, circulation and digestion, few people find the position comfortable or even accessible for any length of time. We have to work with what we've got, so, if you'd like to reclaim the possibility of sitting on the floor, you'll need some props. What we're aiming for is an aligned spine and balance in how we are holding our body. Squatting, kneeling and cross legged poses are safer options. Avoid sitting with your legs swept round to one side: in this position, it is hard to keep the spine erect and shoulders relaxed, and we tend to build asymmetry in strength and flexibility by always twisting to a favoured side.

- **Squatting:** if your hips allow, you could try a squatting posture with your sit bones supported by a bolster, yoga brick or meditation cushion. Be guided by your comfort.

- **Kneeling:** if your knees agree, you could place a bolster between your feet and kneel with your sit bones supported by the bolster. If you need extra height to make this accessible, consider using a stack of several yoga bricks.

- **Cross legged:** if your knees and hips allow, you could come into a cross legged position, seated on a bolster. To protect your lower back, your knees need to be lower than your hips, so add as much height as needed beneath you to facilitate this. If your knees don't reach the floor, place a rolled towel or cushion beneath them for support. Remember we're aiming for balance, so change the cross of your legs so you spend an equal duration of time with each leg in front.

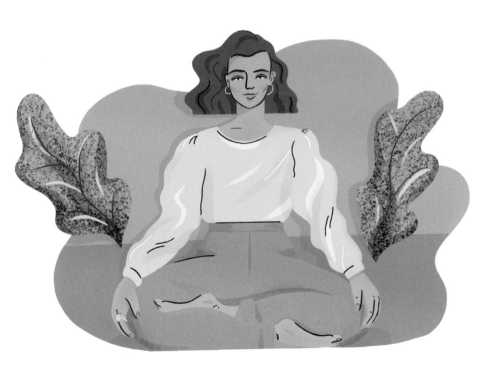

Your
28-day plan

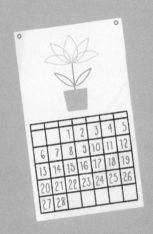

Follow this 28-day plan to develop self-insight, improve your posture, reduce sedentary periods and infuse more movement and restorative practices into your day. We'll use waves of change to help you gradually integrate these new behaviours, making them a pattern you can sustain for the long term. Think of this plan as a new healthy way of sitting and moving through your day from start to finish, with concrete action steps, prompts to check in with your progress and check lists you can tick to record and recognize the commitment you're making. This is how we track behaviour change and boost our motivation.

As you move through the plan, you'll create new rhythm and structure to your day. There will be many nourishing opportunities, so if you miss one, it's ok; take comfort in knowing there'll be another chance soon. Every day we face different demands on our time and energy, but your new toolkit will help you to find effective ways to take care of your health regardless.

There is flexibility in this plan. Different things appeal to different people, so there are options to explore. Try them all, or pick and choose, it's up to you. You can embrace a new focus each day, creating real change in just 28 days, or spend as long as you like on each practice, integrating it into your life before moving on to the next. The aim is a long-term commitment to new habits, so go at your own pace. This is how you'll live your life moving forward.

THE FIVE KEY HEALTHY HABITS OF THE 28-DAY PLAN

○ Morning routine: a practice to start the day with presence and zest in as little as 2 minutes.

○ Daily daylight awe walk: a commitment of at least 5 minutes to boost your mood and help you meet your daily movement target.

○ Micro-moment activities that can be done while seated – think of these as "deskercise" – stretches, self-massage, movements and breathing practices that take less than a minute each.

○ Movement breaks: exercises to counteract the effects of sitting – building muscle strength, promoting circulation and releasing tension – in just a few minutes a day.

○ Evening wind-down rituals: your 5-minute practice to close the day, soothing away stress, aiding digestion and paving the way for deeper sleep.

Day 1.
Get to know yourself

Welcome to your plan of action! Before we embark on any change, we need to connect with personal motivations and get to know ourselves. As we journey through this 28 days together, it will be helpful to jot down observations and any commitments you'd like to make. So your challenge for today is to identify a place to keep this information. It might be a file with loose paper, a journal, or you could use electronic methods. Choose what feels resonant and motivating to you. These notes will help create a feeling of ownership and accountability, allow you to see your progress, and help you to identify behaviour patterns. You might also consider tracking devices, apps or websites (such as Strava or mapometer. com) which can give you feedback on daily sitting time and movement, but these are not essential.

Begin your notes with a check in on your current lifestyle choices, establishing a baseline for later comparison. Jot down how a regular day looks for you right now: how long you sit for, where and how you sit, how often you move and the kind of movement you engage in. It will also be useful to jot down observations about your health and well-being in general. You might choose to record areas of physical pain or tension, you could describe your memory or ability to focus, energy levels, stress levels, mood, the quality of your sleep, digestion and elimination, or self-confidence. Use this information to become more conscious of your current choices and their consequences.

Now you've got to know yourself and recorded your baseline, think about what you'd like to achieve in this plan. Change is challenging for us humans, so articulating why it is important to you is a vital part of the process.

Setting your goals

Read through the Research Round-up chapter (see pages 14–19) on the consequences of sitting, and sitting poorly, and the links between inactivity, posture and well-being. What do you want to avoid and what do you want to achieve? What will motivate you to do things differently? Thinking about why these things are important to you is the key to behaviour change. You don't have to care about "exercise", but you need to treasure what movement and good posture bring to your life, so give it some thought.

For our goals to work, they need to be clear and anchored in what we want for ourselves (rather than in what someone else wants for us). The words we use make a difference too. We are motivated more by goals that are framed positively, stating what we want to do more of, rather than do less of, or avoid. For example, a goal to watch less TV will prime our brains to crave the comfort of a brain fade on the sofa. A goal to roll out your mat for some pre-bedtime yoga, on the other hand, primes your brain for what you *do* want.

Be clear about what you want to achieve. Do you want to move more, improve your posture, reclaim your flexibility, make choices that promote better sleep, boost your energy, develop your ability to stay calm, or create more freedom and ease in your lower back or in your neck and shoulders? If you want to lift your mood, there is some galvanizing recent research showing that movement not only alleviates depression but also protects you from developing it in the future[26]. Exercising for just 20 minutes a day can cut your risk of developing depression by one-third[27]. Jot down in your journal any changes you want to see and get ready to make a tangible, lasting change in your life and your body.

As you move through the plan, write down the action you are taking, documenting your progress. Jot down obstacles that come up too, and proactively brainstorm ways to overcome them. You could put a cross on a calendar on the days you hit your movement or relaxation targets, and that run of crosses will fuel your staying power. In your journal you could write a letter to yourself, reminding you of how good you feel after you've moved or stretched or rested, helping you make that healthy choice again in the future. Keep your journal by your bed or stick your goals up on your refrigerator to keep this commitment fresh in your mind. Say your goals out loud, too, or team up with some friends, so you can motivate each other. Well done for making a start! I look forward to sharing this journey with you.

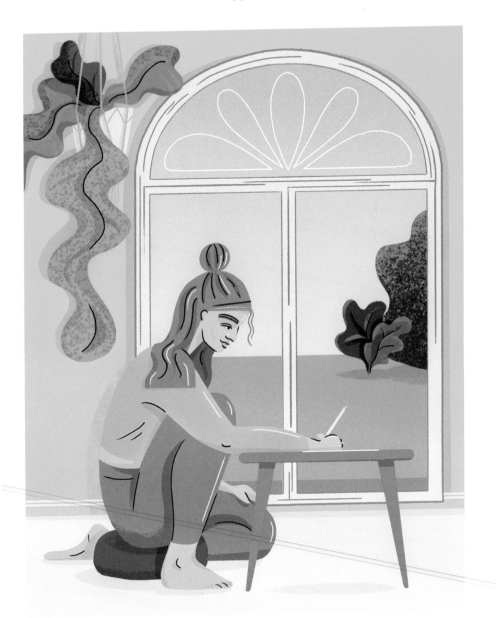

I want to...

- Lift my mood

- Feel energized to play with my children at the end of the working day

- Have restful sleep

- Create a clear separation between working time and downtime

• Enjoy time outside catching up with friends

• Improve my flexibility to feel lighter throughout the day

• Focus my concentration to work more effectively

Day 2.
Introducing your daily morning routine: Mountain Breaths

To begin your day with zest, presence and good posture, welcome to "mountain breaths", your new daily morning routine. This will take as little as a couple of minutes, but its impact can last the whole day long.

Stand tall with your feet hip-width apart, arms down by your sides and gaze forward. Notice how it feels to be standing: the sensation of your feet against the floor, the strength of your legs and core, the elongation of your spine and the buoyancy of your head. You might like to re-read Posture 101 for more cues on creating a feeling of being grounded and tall (see pages 26–45). Now begin moving with your breath, where you will breathe in and out through your nose unless you are congested. On your next inhalation slowly raise your arms out to your sides and up above your head, looking up to your hands, palms touching when you finish breathing in. Allow a tiny pause here and then enjoy a long, slow exhalation, gazing forward again, palms reaching your outer thighs when you are ready to finish breathing out.

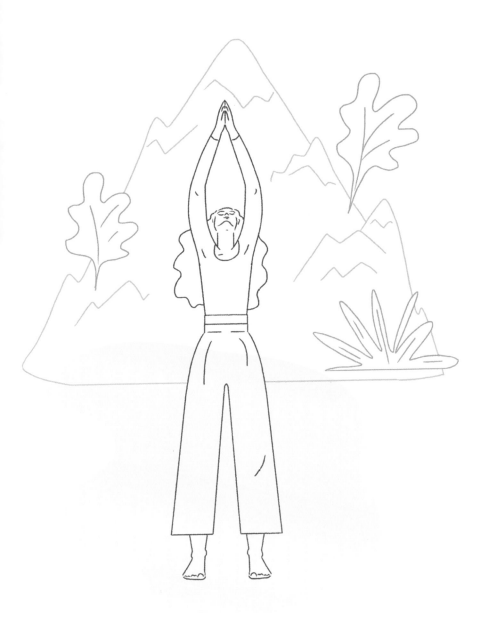

Repeat this mindful movement in time with your breath 5–10 times. Feel how this sequence helps you lift more effortlessly into good posture. Not only are you waking up to the day, you are waking up your mindfulness muscles, helping you become more aware of your body and breath.

Once this sequence feels comfortable, we're going to pair it with a breathing practice called coherent breathing. The goal with this is to breathe at a rate of 6 breaths per minute, which means we inhale for 5 seconds and exhale for 5 seconds. This brings the lungs and heart into synchrony and is soothing for your nervous system[28]. The "mountain breath" exercise lends itself beautifully to this ratio of breathing, and, by pairing the 2 activities, we are not only developing better posture but also re-patterning our breathing. Coherent breathing is something you can return to at any interval in your day to create a feeling of calm, either including the "mountain breath" arm movement or on its own. Together they are the perfect alternative to a caffeine hit – your adrenal glands will be grateful and you'll notice a better quality of sleep, too.

You choose when to engage in this morning ritual. It could be the first thing you do as your feet hit the floor after getting out of bed. You might prefer to do it after your shower, or perhaps right before you begin your working day. Earmark a time that fits naturally in your day and make it a daily feature, as potent and treasured as your morning coffee, setting you up for your day. Aim to do this routine every day, ticking off the check box every day you do.

In embarking on this morning routine, you are building your ability to notice your body, patterns of tension, time spent sitting, your posture and your breath. To further bring this wakeful quality to your whole day, identify salient opportunities to check in with yourself. It could be while brushing your teeth, during your shower, when you first sit down at your desk, while stopped at a red light, during bathroom breaks, while the kettle is boiling, while sending emails, checking social media or when you receive a message notification. If you need to at first, set a timer to remind yourself to notice your posture, mood, energy or mental clarity and anywhere there is tension. Then take a moment to loosen up your body, lift your spirits or boost your concentration. See what grows from your newfound awareness and jot it down in your journal.

○ Morning routine

Day 3.
Environment review:
seated set-ups

Scan your environment and identify all the places you regularly sit, lie down or recline – in your home, in your car, on your bike and while working. Use the healthy sitting guidelines in Posture 101 (see pages 26–45) to evaluate each of these set-ups. Remember that good ergonomics do not negate the harmful effects of being sedentary – even with the perfect set-up, we still need to get up and move every 30 minutes – but do look for ways that you can make yourself more comfortable. Make the necessary adjustments or investments you need to protect your health now. Don't wait for pain to be the catalyst, which is likely to be more costly than taking swift preventative action.

Don't forget where you spend your leisure time, especially while watching TV or scrolling on your phone. Think of simple ways you can support the natural curve of your spine and your joints, such as a rolled-up blanket underneath your knees if your legs are outstretched, or a cushion behind the small of your back. Watch out for sinking sofas: if you have zippered base cushions, you can combat sagging with foam inserts, or it might be time to consider an upgrade. Or commit to your unwinding practices and make sitting on the floor a viable option at least some of the time. Don't even try to optimize your bed for sitting upright. If you want to read in bed, lie on your side, or lie back supported by a "V"-shaped pillow. Avoid taking work to bed – you want to have a strong association between bed and sleep, not bed and a "to do" list, and sitting in bed while using your devices is a sure-fire way both to create tension and diminish the quality of rest.

○ Morning routine

Day 4.
Introducing your
micro-moments

These are 60-second rituals that you can perform while sitting at your computer or on the sofa.

SHRUG AND SIGH

Feeling the weight of the world on your shoulders? Reclaim your neck by making tight fists with your hands, at the same time squeezing your shoulders up to your ears and wrinkling your face into a tiny raisin. Now let it all go with a cathartic sigh, allowing the day to drop off your shoulders.

PROTECT YOUR PEACE

Bring your hands to rest across your heart, feeling their warmth and the beating of your heart beneath them. Close your eyes and let the world wait for you. Take a few calming breaths into your hands, feeling your heart centre expand with the inhalation, releasing what you no longer need with your exhalation. Blink your eyes open and re-enter your day with peaceful poise, knowing you can come back to this calm place whenever you need.

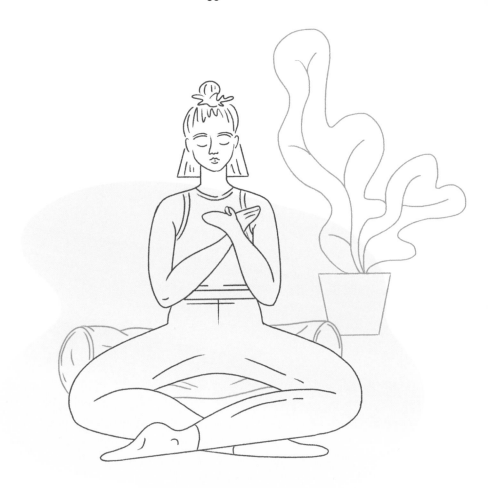

○ Morning routine

○ Micro-moment

Day 5.
Developing your
movement mindset

Today your challenge is to identify alternatives to sitting during the rhythm of your daily life and ways that you can use your environment to prompt you to move. Often, when we are confronted with the possibility of sitting, we don't even see other options... so the other half of the battle is remembering! Grab your journal and jot down some simple swaps for activities you normally do seated, or ways you can tailor your environment to encourage more movement. Here are some ideas to consider:

- Stand while you talk on the phone, or during Zoom calls.

- Schedule walking meetings.

- Stand and record a voice note rather than sitting to text or email.

- Meet a friend for a takeaway coffee and walk together.

- Take a brainstorming session out into nature's beauty.

- Bring your ironing board into the living room and stand and iron while watching the TV.

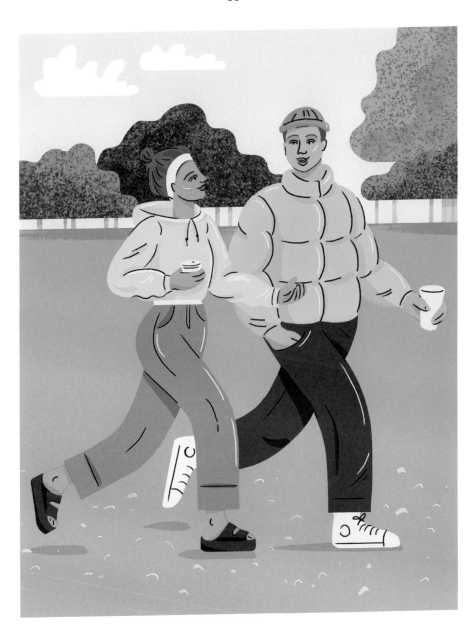

- Use a small glass that you need to get up to fill rather than keeping a large bottle at your desk. You could even create a habit of standing up when you hydrate yourself.

- Move your printer away from your desk set-up so you have to move to use it.

- Keep a yoga mat out on the living-room floor and have a gentle stretch to relax, rather than habitually slumping on the sofa.

- Wear a posture biofeedback device to remind you to sit upright.

- Set a reminder on your phone to prompt you to move every 30 minutes.

- Find an accountability buddy and drop each other messages during the day, reminding each other to move. Check in at agreed intervals to provide support and to offer encouragement.

- Use TV advertising breaks as a reminder to move.

- Leave yourself notes in key locations around the house with relevant inspiration – in the bathroom, remind yourself of your "seated spine twist" and "tummy rubs" (see page 116). Keep a mind map or visual diagram of soothing practices by your bed, standing movement inspiration on the refrigerator, a list of seated stretches and joint mobilizations by the sofa. Affix a note of self-massage and breathing exercises to your computer.

- Strategically place items to prompt action – walking boots by your front door, your journal by your bed, hand weights in the living room, resistance band and eye pillow by the sofa, therapy ball by your desk... and this book right next to your mouse.

- Mentally pair everyday activities with movement rituals – while you're waiting for the microwave to ping, folding the washing or stacking the dishwasher. Notice the impulse to check in with social media? Move before you scroll, and, once you've had your fix, rest your senses with a calming practice.

Make a mind map of all the ways you enjoy moving your body – think laterally, not just of exercise or sport, but of any joyful movement. Make a note of any exercise classes you might like, to take it one step further – and make time for it! Put it in the diary. Enlist a friend to help you make it happen.

○ Morning routine

○ Micro-moment

Day 6.
Introducing your daily daylight awe walk

Your challenge for today is to take a daylight walk, with the express intention of leaving your worries at home, and train your eyes to seek out anything awe-inspiring. To minimize distraction, leave your phone at home, pop it on silent or switch it to aeroplane mode. Head out, look up and see what you can see! It might be wildlife, plant life, shadows, intriguing architecture or inspiration you glean from connecting with other people out and about. Research shows that taking an awe walk boosts our health and well-being[29] and so we hit two birds with a single stone, simultaneously building our mood-boosting mindfulness muscles and helping us hit our daily movement target. Take that walk somewhere green and you will also receive the potent anti-depressant effect of nature's beauty.

Head out during daylight and get your daily dose of natural light, regulating your circadian rhythms and helping you to sleep better at night. For so many reasons, your daylight awe walk is a powerful ritual. When you get home, you might like to put pen to paper, describing how your walk felt, what you noticed while out, and the walk's impact on your well-being throughout the rest of your day. These little letters to yourself can be useful primers for repeating healthy action down the track, and we all need reminding of that every now and then.

If it resonates for you, identify a window of time to take this daylight awe walk daily. If it is a new habit, start small. Grand, elaborate plans are hard to sustain, and we know that even small bouts of movement are beneficial. Think of the duration of time that feels genuinely achievable, knowing that you can build on this as your stamina develops or time allows. As little as 5 minutes is enough to clear your head and see the benefits. Over time, gradually build up to 20 minutes daily. If you are already accustomed to heading out regularly, add the skill of awe to the exercise and feel how this gives you an extra boost. Even incidental trips out, such as zipping to the post office, can be transformed when we see them through the lens of awe.

Let's be honest, even with activities we enjoy, it can be hard to make a habit stick. It is genuinely challenging to make the healthy choice over the easy one. So, to avoid the "will I... won't I?" dilemma, we need some concrete strategies. My first suggestion is to make an "appointment" with yourself, protecting the time you choose so it is more likely to happen. If you keep it at the same time each day, you reduce the number of choices you need to make, and, again, you're more likely to take the nourishing action. You will find that the appointment becomes a non-negotiable moment, like brushing your teeth. Earlier in the day is preferable, because our decision-making capacity is likely to be higher in the morning, we will get the benefits for

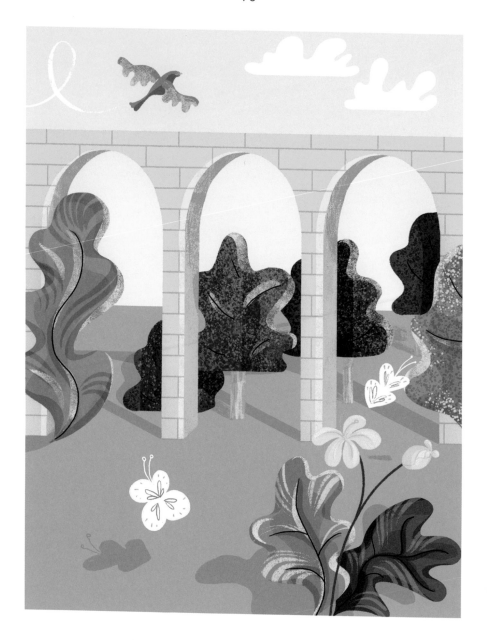

longer and it tends to create a cascading effect of other healthier choices. Setting the intention to do it daily is another helpful strategy – if you aim for three times a week, it is easier to put it off until tomorrow, or the next day, or the next. Make the commitment daily, there's less quibbling that way and it is an easier habit to form. You may wish to set different intentions for weekdays and weekend days, or to match other variations in your week.

Plan ahead and make this habit your own. If you'd rather pick a different daily habit, by all means do so! The choice is yours. Every day you engage in your daily movement habit, pop a cross on your calendar and soon that run of crosses will provide juicy motivation to keep you going. Life will inevitably throw you curveballs though, so don't worry if you miss a day. If you can't get out, you could always switch it up for an indoor sequence, and, if energy is low, opt for a soothing stretching practice instead. Take your time building this habit. Don't feel any pressure to instigate more change until this habit is ingrained in everyday life.

○ Morning routine

○ Micro-moment

○ Daily daylight awe walk

Day 7.
Introducing your evening wind-down ritual

Today we're embarking on a new ritual to release tension and revitalize, perfect to close the day. Ideally we'd invest 5 minutes, but if that feels like too much right now, the ritual can be as simple as a single relaxation pose. Just like the morning routine (see page 56), our aim is to do this daily. You could also use this ritual to navigate that very common post-lunch energy lull, or when you're sleep deprived.

SQUEEZE AND RELEASE

If you find it hard to relax your body, this activity will help you to cultivate the skill. This sequence uses the strategy of gentle exertion to encourage a deep physical letting go. Lie down on the floor, knees bent, feet flat on the floor, hip-width apart. Place your palms flat on your thighs and let your head relax completely. Make sure your head is cushioned by either lying on a yoga mat or placing a folded blanket under your head. As you breathe in, let your whole body relax. As you breathe out, press your hands down into your thighs and your feet down into the floor. Soften your hands and feet as you breathe in, and again powerfully ground them with each exhalation. Notice that by pressing your hands and feet down, your core muscles leap into action. Don't try to engage them, just focus your attention on your hands and feet and keep your head on the floor throughout. Do 10 repetitions and notice how much easier it is to relax your body after some mild exertion. Release your spine at the end, by drawing your knees to your chest.

RESTING POSE

Stretch your legs out long, feet hip-width apart, and let your toes drop out to the sides. Bring your arms to rest, palms facing upward a little away from your sides. Aim to bring your body to symmetry, closing your eyes, head well-cushioned, sinking into the floor. Give yourself permission to let go. We spend all day holding ourselves up, now is the time to flop and drop. The beauty of this resting pose is that it realigns the spine, releases your postural muscles and builds your relaxation skills. Enjoy the absence of effort, letting gravity do the work for you, feeling how this is the perfect counterbalance to all the activity and stimulation of your day. Become well practised at this exercise and notice how much easier sleep comes when you finally do hop into bed.

If there is any discomfort in your lower back or knees, you can either place a rolled-up blanket or a cushion underneath your knees, or bend your knees and place your feet flat on the floor. Be guided by your body, knowing we don't want to skimp on comfort here.

Pop on an eye pillow or mask, wrap yourself up in a weighted blanket and drop. If your mind feels busy, anchor it on the sensation of your body releasing to the floor, or count out your breath using your coherent breathing ratio of 5 seconds in and 5 seconds out (see page 58). An alternative is to seek out a guided version of this resting pose, known as "savasana" in yoga.

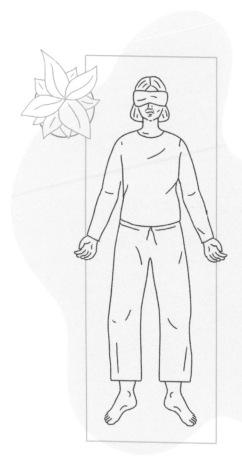

○ Morning routine

○ Micro-moment

○ Daily daylight awe walk

○ Evening wind down

WEEKLY CHECK IN

We're 7 days in...Well done! What action have you taken so far?

Recognize your accomplishments, big and small. Notice the fruits of your labour. It's not just physical results we are after.

- Are you noticing any changes in your mood or energy levels?

- Are there any changes in your stress levels or the quality of your sleep?

- How are you doing with building your awareness?

Your mindfulness muscles are just as important as your core muscles. Reward your efforts as well as celebrating progress! Jot down in your journal any tweaks to your goals, or write encouraging notes to your future self.

Day 8.
Introducing your
movement inspiration

This is a standing exercise to strengthen your legs and get the blood pumping.

TAI CHI SUMO SQUAT

Stand with your feet one and half times your shoulder-width apart, toes angled out. Breathe in, and, as you exhale, bend your knees deeply in the same direction as your toes and press your hands firmly forward like two stop signs. As you breathe in, slowly straighten your legs, turning your palms to face you and drawing your hands toward your chest. Repeat this slow, mindful squatting 10 times, keeping your spine tall and your gaze forward. As you squat and your hands press away, imagine releasing what no longer serves you and, as you straighten your legs and bring your hands back in, imagine you're drawing in fresh energy. Extra challenge: try lifting your toes! This makes it harder to balance, but might also engage more core muscles – the same ones you are learning to switch on in the "squeeze and release" exercise in your evening ritual (see page 72).

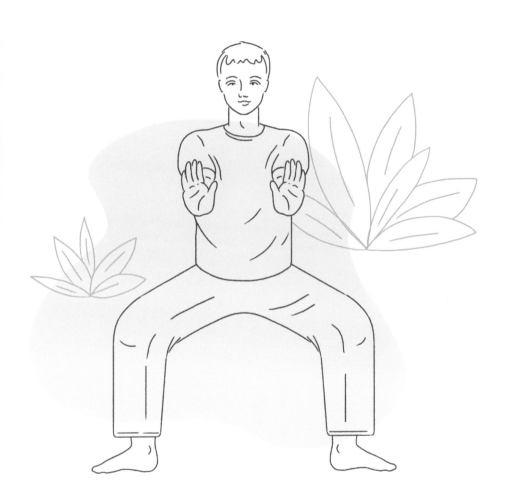

HULA HOOP HIPS

Bring your feet to hip-width apart, knees generously bent, hands on hips and imagine you are spinning a giant hula hoop around your waist. Making the action as large as possible, feel this "oil" the hips and bring your stomach muscles to life. After 6 loops in each direction, give your legs a good shake out.

SUMO SIDE BENDS

Come back to your "tai chi sumo squat" stance (see page 76), but this time stay in it: the deeper the knee bend, the greater the challenge. Hovering in your squat, inhale and stretch your arms out to shoulder height, then exhale and reach your left arm up and over, right arm rounded loosely in front and banana-shaping the whole left-hand side of your torso. Breathe in and come back to the centre with your arms wide like wings, exhale, then lift your right arm up and over, left arm rounded in front of your body, arching your right-hand side. Inhale back to the centre. Alternate the bend, 3–6 times each way.

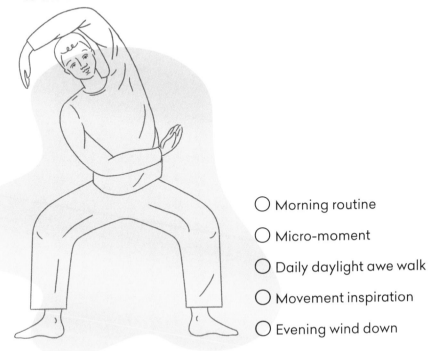

○ Morning routine

○ Micro-moment

○ Daily daylight awe walk

○ Movement inspiration

○ Evening wind down

Day 9.
Growing your morning routine: intention setting

Before you take your morning "mountain breaths" (see page 56), think of one quality that's important to you, something that might help you navigate your day, such as patience, curiosity or kindness. Breathe life into this intention with your 5–10 "mountain breaths", further developing your mindfulness muscles and deepening the practice with a sense of purpose. You can just think about how it feels to embody this quality, or you could repeat your intention like a mantra. For example, on the inhalation, repeat "*I am*" and on the exhalation repeat "*calm*". Think about an everyday action that you can use to check in with this intention. Drinking a tall glass of water provides an excellent opportunity to reaffirm your commitment and fine-tune your presence of mind.

If you'd like to also add a new physical element to this practice, roll up a towel and place it between your thighs. You may need to bring your feet a little narrower than hip-width to keep the towel in place. Take your "mountain breaths" while gently squeezing the towel and feel how this engages your thighs and deep lower abdominal muscles. Enjoy how this develops not only your awareness of your core but also your ability to recruit those muscles and feel well supported.

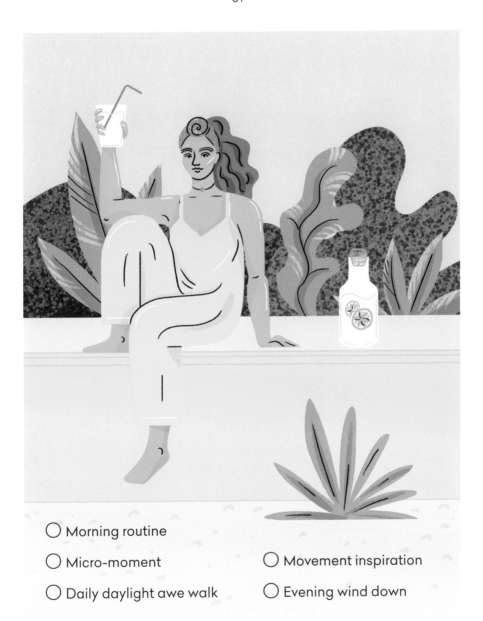

○ Morning routine

○ Micro-moment   ○ Movement inspiration

○ Daily daylight awe walk   ○ Evening wind down

Day 10.
Environment review:
sleep zone

It's not just our seated and standing postures that impact our well-being, the position you sleep in is important, too. If you're waking up with achey shoulders, a crick in the neck or a sore lower back, you might need to check your sleep environment and sleeping posture.

While there are no hard-and-fast features of the perfect mattress, the best type for you is one that helps you feel comfortable and well supported and allows you to wake with no soreness. Check the state of your mattress: look for signs of wear, and flip or rotate it if need be. Ideally mattresses should be replaced every 10 years and your pillow every year. Your pillow should support the natural curve of your neck, keeping your head level with your spine, so this may vary according to the position you sleep in. Front sleepers might need a very flat pillow, or prefer to dispense with one under the head entirely.

Different sleeping positions have different benefits, and ultimately what is best for you will depend on what feels most comfortable to you. Lying on your back with your spine well supported protects your lower back, hips and knees, but can exacerbate snoring and sleep apnoea.

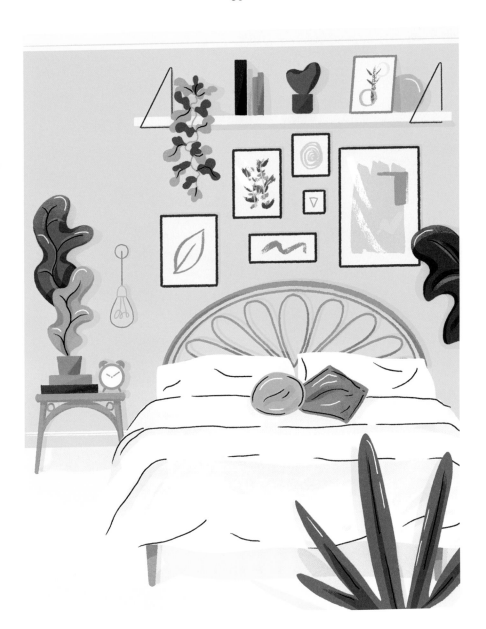

Side lying can be a good option, but make sure you are well supported to avoid discomfort in your shoulders. Be wary of sleeping on your stomach, which can cause neck and back pain. Depending on your sleep posture, extra pillows can help keep your spine aligned. If you sleep on your back, you might benefit from a pillow beneath your knees. Side sleepers might find more comfort with a pillow between their knees (it's best to aim for a gentle bend in the knees rather than hugging them in tight) and experiment with embracing a pillow to support their chest and arms. For front sleepers, placing a pillow under the lower abdomen can reduce back pain. Be mindful of changing position in bed too, avoiding jerky twisting movements and turning your body as one unit in alignment. Crisp, clean sheets can promote calmer, deeper sleep, too.

Consider where you take your naps. It's better not to drop off on a squishy sofa with your head lolling about. Feeling dozy? Get an early night, or, if it's daytime, set yourself up on the floor in your "resting pose" from Day 7 (see page 73). If you're on a hard floor you'll need a yoga mat, rug or folded blanket beneath you. Make sure you have a pillow supporting your head and another beneath your knees, drape yourself with a blanket and pop on an eye pillow for maximum comfort. Drift off in a position that promotes circulation and helps to realign the spine. You might have to set yourself a gentle-sounding alarm!

Growing your evening ritual

If you'd like a new soothing pose to try, or an alternative to your lying "resting pose" on Day 7 (see page 73), try "child's pose" (see below). The choice is yours, just keep taking some kind of soothing action before bed.

CHILD'S POSE

Begin on all fours, with your knees hip-width apart, big toes touching. Slide your bottom to your heels and bring your forearms and forehead to the floor. If your head doesn't comfortably reach the floor, rest it on your folded hands, make a fist or stack both fists on top of each other and rest your head on that. Sink into this shape, feeling the pleasant sensation of "earthing your brow". Stay for 10 breaths, longer if it feels good.

○ Morning routine

○ Micro-moment

○ Daily daylight awe walk

○ Movement inspiration

○ Evening wind down

Day 11.
Micro-moments:
releasing tech stress

RECLAIM YOUR NECK

Make a few head turns to "oil" your neck. Keeping your jaw parallel to the floor, gaze right, then gaze left. Next, draw a "U" shape with your chin. Start with your chin to your chest, then loll your chin toward your right shoulder, back down to your chest and over to your left shoulder. Repeat a few times to each side. Finish with your chin dropping heavily to your chest for a few calm breaths.

SOOTHE YOUR EYES

Vigorously rub your hands together to create heat. Close your eyes and place your palms over your eyes so that the fingertips cup your head. Feel the warmth penetrate and soothe the muscles of your eyes and enjoy the absence of stimulation. Relish several soothing breaths here before releasing and re-entering your day.

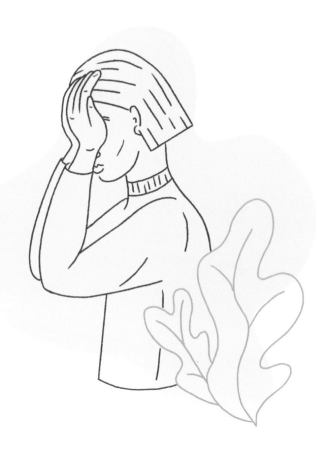

○ Morning routine

○ Micro-moment

○ Daily daylight awe walk

○ Movement inspiration

○ Evening wind down

Day 12. Growing your decision-making power: constructive self-talk

Contrary to what you've been led to believe, being tough on yourself seldom helps you to make healthier choices. When it comes to healthy habits, we are constantly faced with choices... do I sit and slob out on the sofa, or do I take that walk I had planned? Do I plough on with this report, or do I get up and take a few stretches? Move over inner critic! Research shows that self-forgiveness helps you regulate your behaviour and opt for the healthy choice more often[30].

So, as we move through this plan, watch your inner dialogue. Know that you can choose kinder, coaxing words and this not only makes all the difference to your energy, mood and self-esteem, but will help you make these concrete lifestyle changes. A neat little trick, again backed by research[31], is to refer to yourself by your name or a pet name. When we address ourselves by our names, we are naturally more tender and compassionate. Use "I" and it tends to follow with something more punitive. When you fall short of your expectations, use encouraging words, forgive yourself and reaffirm your commitment to your path of action. It is challenging to make change. Permission to be human? Granted.

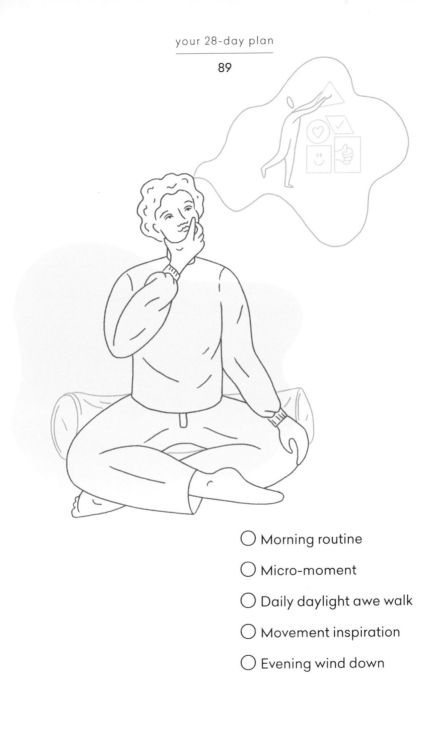

○ Morning routine

○ Micro-moment

○ Daily daylight awe walk

○ Movement inspiration

○ Evening wind down

Day 13.
Environment review:
mindful decoration

Lift your line of sight by purposefully placing art or images up high at key focal points around your home, lifting you more effortlessly into an upright posture. Set the intention to gaze on these, giving yourself permission to refresh with a micro break. Pop a vase of cut flowers or a houseplant by your desk. When concentration flags, zoom in on them, remembering that sometimes rest is the most productive choice possible.

○ Morning routine

○ Micro-moment

○ Daily daylight awe walk

○ Movement inspiration

○ Evening wind down

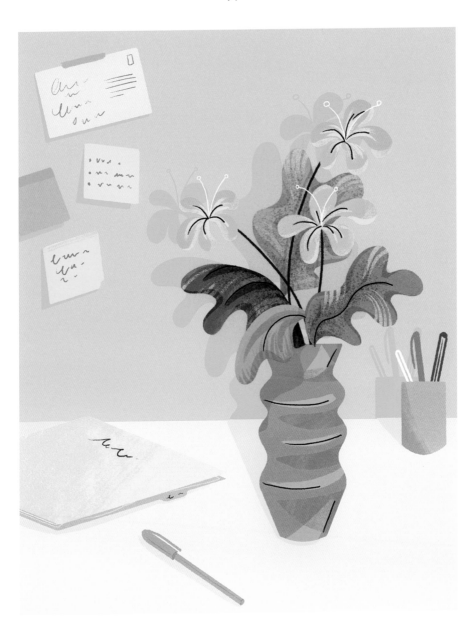

Day 14.
Movement breaks:
spring clean!

Remember, it's not just "exercise" that counts, incidental movement does too. You can use everyday action as an antidote to sitting, as well. Reframe household tasks from drudgery into "moving for mental health" – folding the washing, DIY, vacuuming, dusting, mopping, sweeping, blitzing the bathroom, making the beds, making mash... and you can't beat gardening for all its squatting and bending. Up the inspiration and pair these tasks with music, podcasts or an audio book to engage your senses. Make a menu of everyday household activities that you can use to get your movement quota up and notice how it can invigorate you.

○ Morning routine

○ Micro-moment

○ Daily daylight awe walk

○ Movement inspiration

○ Evening wind down

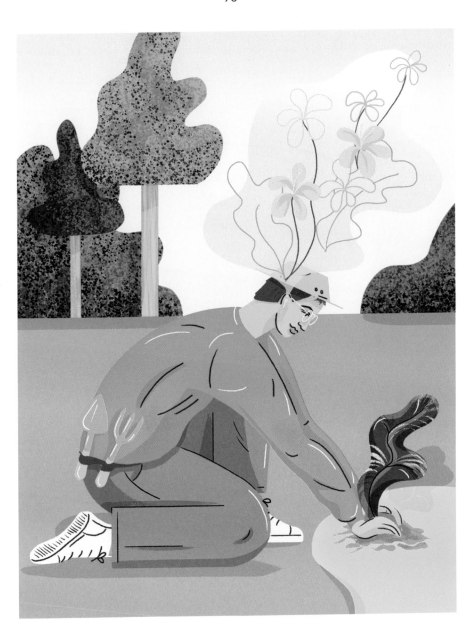

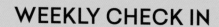

WEEKLY CHECK IN

Give yourself a pat on the back! You are halfway through your 28 days. Take a moment to check in with your progress. Recognize the actions you have taken and see them all for the true accomplishments they are.

- **Of your new daily habits, what's working best for you?**

- **Is there a habit that needs more attention?**

- **What changes are you noticing?**

Remember, the change we are aiming for is long term, so small and steady is the goal. Go gently as you integrate these new ways of moving through your day. And remember your kind and coaxing self-talk (see page 88).

Day 15.
Wind-down inspiration:
free your hips

How to sit like a monk... try this sequence as part of your evening wind-down ritual (see page 72), or whenever fatigue hits. These powerful hip openers are perfect for people who spend much of their day sitting, freeing up the body to return to a more natural sitting position such as cross legged on the floor, squatting or kneeling.

JOINT WARM-UPS

Sit on the floor with your legs outstretched, feet shoulder-width apart, hands on the floor behind you for support. Limber your ankle joints by circling your feet, 5 rotations in each direction. Point and flex your feet, again 5 times each way. "Windscreen-wiper" your feet, by swishing your toes out to the sides and then toward each other, letting the whole leg oscillate with the movement. Finish off with a gentle alternating bounce of the knees. You now feel warm, connected and your legs are released from the constraints of the day.

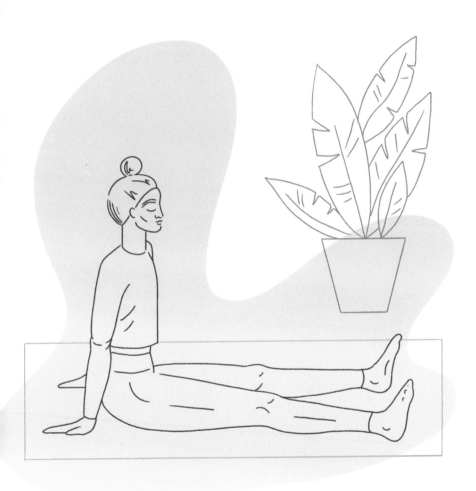

SEATED KNEE HUG TWIST

Bend your right knee, keeping the sole of the foot flat on the floor, and stretch your left leg straight in front of you, heel flexed. Hug your left arm around your right knee and, as you breathe in, raise your right arm skyward. As you exhale, twist to the right, bringing your right hand to the floor behind you, gazing deeply over your right shoulder. Sit tall in the twist for 5–10 breaths before releasing and repeating on the other side.

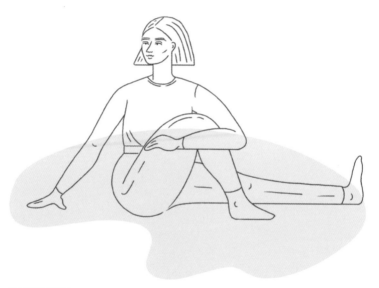

BUTTERFLY

Bend both knees and bring the soles of your feet to touch. Walk your hands forward and, without force, drop your chin to your chest. Hang out in your effortless fold for 5–10 breaths, letting your knees drop heavily.

SWAN TWIST

From "butterfly", tuck your right leg back behind you with the knee bent, right knee touching the sole of your left foot. Take a regal, upright twist to the left, bringing your right hand to your left knee and your left fingertips to the floor behind you. Lift your heart, pin your inner right knee to the floor like an anchor and gaze over your left shoulder. Relish the stretch in the front of your right thigh and the release through the side of your body. Take 5–10 breaths in this refreshing twist before unravelling your legs and repeating on the other side.

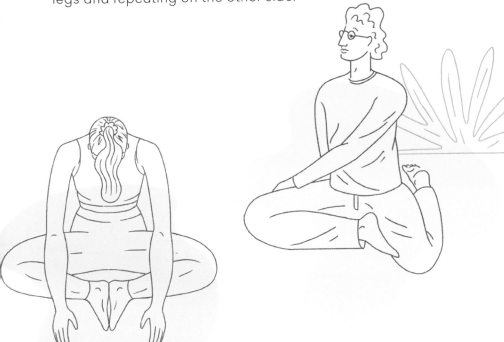

BUTTOCK STRETCH

From "butterfly", bring your left leg back behind you so it's out of the way. Flex your right heel and make a right angle with your right knee. Bring one hand either side of your right knee and foot and, bending your elbows, lower your chest toward your right shin. Keep your right heel flexed and your hips and chest square and feel the release for the muscles of your right hip, the glutes in particular: hello, butt muscles! Take 5–10 slow breaths before repeating with the left leg forward.

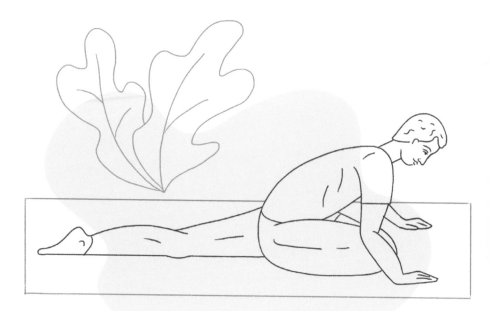

SEATED FOLD

Extending your legs in front of you and keeping your knees bent, reach forward and take hold of whatever you can comfortably touch. It needn't be your toes, your calves are just fine. Breathe in and elongate your spine, stretching the front of your body. Keeping this length, as you exhale, lower your chest toward your knees and your chin toward your shins. Take 5–10 calm breaths here, stretching the back of your entire body. Slowly rise, give your knees a little bounce out again and feel the freedom you've just created in your hips.

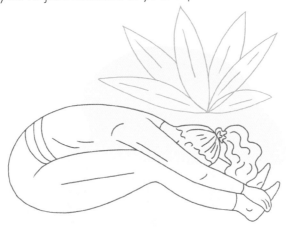

○ Morning routine

○ Micro-moment   ○ Movement inspiration

○ Daily daylight awe walk   ○ Evening wind down

Day 16.
Micro-moments:
free your arms

WRIST RELEASE

Stretch out your hands right to your fingertips and take a flamboyant "flamenco-style" wrist rotation, it's much juicier than doing it with a fist. Take 5 in each direction.

HAND RELEASE

Interlace your hands at chest height in front of you, elongate your arms and press your palms away from you to release the fascia of your palms. The perfect antidote to mouse work. Check in and relax your shoulders and jaw as you take 5 breaths here.

GREET YOUR TRICEPS

Take your right arm skyward and bend the right elbow, keeping it pointing straight up. Either anchor the stretch by taking hold of the right elbow with your left hand or, if the

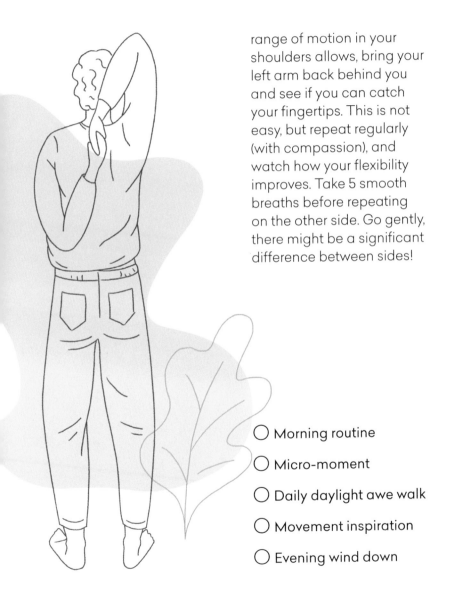

range of motion in your shoulders allows, bring your left arm back behind you and see if you can catch your fingertips. This is not easy, but repeat regularly (with compassion), and watch how your flexibility improves. Take 5 smooth breaths before repeating on the other side. Go gently, there might be a significant difference between sides!

- ○ Morning routine
- ○ Micro-moment
- ○ Daily daylight awe walk
- ○ Movement inspiration
- ○ Evening wind down

Day 17.
Movement breaks: your whole body workout circuit

Complete this circuit 1–3 times.

PRESS-UPS

Choose your press-up: wall, box or the full version. New to press-ups? Take the wall version. Stand a little more than one arm's length away from the wall, feet hip-width apart. Place your palms flat against the wall at shoulder height and a little wider apart than your shoulders. As you breathe in, keeping your spine in neutral position – so no sagging – engage your legs (lift your knee caps up and draw your thigh muscles toward your thigh bones) and lower your body toward the wall. As you exhale, press back to your start position. Move slowly, gently drawing your navel toward your spine throughout, and aim for 10 reps.

The intermediate version is on the floor with the knees grounded. From all fours, hands placed slightly wider than your shoulders, bring your knees just a little further back than your hips and, keeping your spine in neutral with your core engaged as above, slowly lower your torso toward the floor on the inhalation and exhale just as slowly back up.

For an extra challenge, try the full press-up position on your toes. Only take this variation if you can keep your abdominal muscles and thigh muscles engaged throughout. To get maximum support from your legs, press your heels away from you throughout. If you get floppy around the middle, it's better to opt for the kneeling version instead, or try a handful of full press-ups and pop your knees down when you begin to lose your form and carry on to 10 reps. It can be exciting to watch the number grow as your strength develops, objective feedback that things are changing.

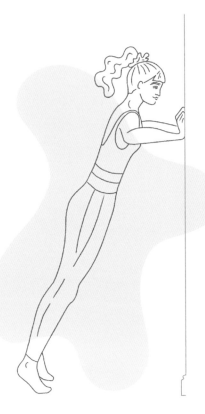

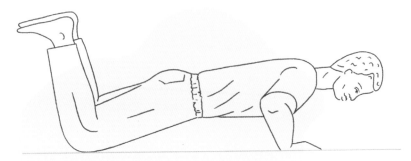

NARROW SQUAT AND ALTERNATING FRONT KICK

Begin standing with your feet hip-width apart, arms bent like a boxer, elbows in, hands in a gentle fist by your ears. Bend your knees, sinking your bottom back behind you into an imaginary chair. The lower you go, the greater the challenge, but let the comfort of your body determine the depth. Straighten your legs and complete a front kick with your right foot, imagining you are striking in front of you with your heel. Ground your right foot again and sink immediately into your squat. Rise back to upright and front kick with your left heel. This sequence has a faster pace to it than your press-ups – squatting on the in breath and pressing your heel into the front kick on the out breath. Keep your hands by your ears, pull your navel to your spine and feel the blood pump! Aim for 5–10 kicks on each leg.

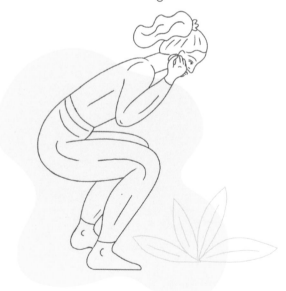

STANDING GLUTE BALANCE

Bring the heart rate back down with this stretch. Take your right ankle across your left thigh, right heel flexed, and lower your right knee toward the floor. Sink into a squat, holding onto a wall – or just a fingertip touch to the wall – for security if needed. If you can go hands free, bring your palms to touch at your heart centre. Hang out here for 5–10 breaths. If there's a little juice left in the tank, add a twist for 5 breaths: take the back of your right hand to your right instep and reach your left arm straight back behind you (easier said than done!), rotating your chest, and gaze toward the left. Feel this powerfully engage the muscles behind your left shoulder; your legs will have something to say about it too. Unravel, shake out your legs and repeat on the other side.

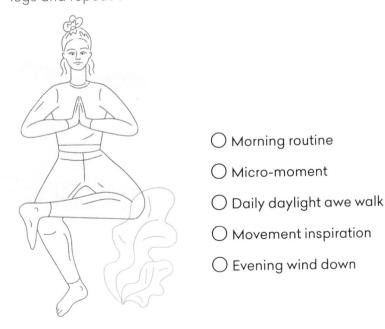

○ Morning routine

○ Micro-moment

○ Daily daylight awe walk

○ Movement inspiration

○ Evening wind down

Day 18.
Micro-moments: time out

GREEN GAZING

Take a break from "up-close" focus and engage in green gazing. Either head to the window, or, if you can see nature from your desk, cast a soft, liquid gaze, enjoying taking in (ideally) the green foliage of trees around you, the cloudscape, or watching out for birds flying by. As you enjoy this nature break, remember to soften your hands, resting them in your lap if you're seated.

HEART OPENER

Interlace your hands behind your back and draw them down toward the floor to stretch your chest wide. Hang out here for a few spacious breaths.

HUG IT OUT

Wrap your arms around yourself to release your upper back. Soften into the stretch by seeing if you can send 3 deep breaths into your fingertips. Repeat with the other arm on top.

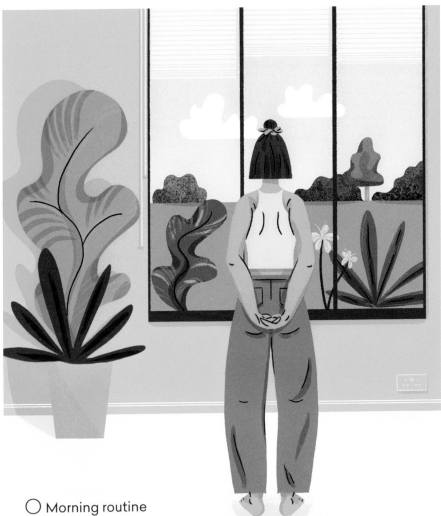

○ Morning routine

○ Micro-moment   ○ Movement inspiration

○ Daily daylight awe walk   ○ Evening wind down

Day 19.
Movement breaks:
core strength

This floor sequence will connect you with the muscles that keep you in your tall, open-hearted posture without even having to think about it.

ALL FOURS WARM-UP

Come to all fours, knees hip-width apart, hands placed a little wider than shoulder-width apart and fingers spread out like starfish. Start with a gentle sway from side to side, preparing your arms for strength work and lubricating your hip joints. Turn the sway into a larger circle, moving your hips around your knees, 5 times in each direction, making the movement as large as feels comfortable for you.

DOG TAIL AND ANGRY CAT

Return to all fours in stillness. As you breathe in, draw your shoulders deeply away from your ears, gaze forward (not up), keeping your neck long and raise your doggy tail high to the sky. This shape stretches the

front of your body and strengthens your back. As you
exhale, bring your chin to your chest, draw your navel to
your spine and point your tailbone to the floor in angry
cat shape. This position elongates the back of your
body and strengthens your stomach muscles. Alternate
between these 2 shapes, led by your breathing, and
repeat 5 times each.

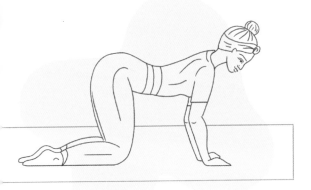

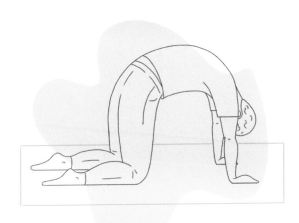

COBRA

Lower your body to rest on the floor, legs together, toes pointing back behind you. Place your hands directly below your shoulders with the fingers splayed wide, elbows pointing straight back behind you. Inhale in this resting position. As you exhale, press firmly into your hands, peeling just your chest away from the floor, gazing downward to keep the back of your neck long. You can activate your legs by pressing the tops of your feet into the floor, but keep your buttocks soft. The movement in Cobra is small (but the effort can feel intense, so work at your own pace) – we are not aiming to lift the stomach off the floor and your arms will remain bent, elbows pinned by your side. Keep lifting on the exhale and releasing on the inhale, 5–10 times. Enjoy a well-deserved rest, lying on your tummy if this is comfortable to you, or come into "child's pose" (see page 85) and release the muscles you have just exerted.

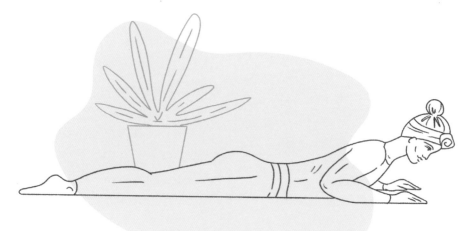

DYNAMIC QUADRUPED

Return to all fours, but get ready to balance. As you inhale, reach your right arm out in front of you and stretch your left leg back behind you. As you exhale, sweep your right arm back behind you, bringing your left knee and chin toward each other. Inhale and reach out, exhale and repeat the round spine movement. Take 5–10 repetitions on this side before changing limbs. Finish with a rest pose of your choice, front lying or "child's pose" (see page 85).

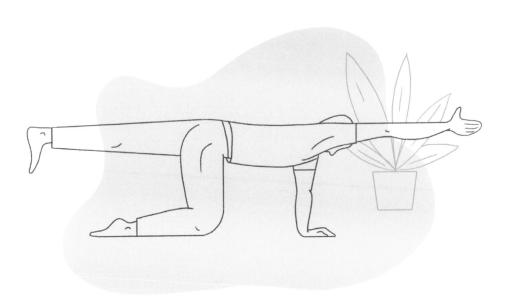

DOWNWARD DOG WITH A TWIST!

From all fours, tuck your toes under, lift up your hips and press your heels back and down. Our goal here is to elongate the spine and work the muscles of your arms and shoulders. We achieve this better by having a gentle bend in the knee. Don't be overly concerned about working the legs straight to feel that powerful hamstring stretch that is often the goal of this shape. Now for the twist – to activate your rhomboids, the muscles that hold your shoulder blades flat to your back, spin your fingertips to point out to the sides, rather than the usual placement of pointing forward. Feel how this instantly draws your shoulders away from your ears, lengthening your neck. Stay here for 5 breaths, focusing on the engagement of these muscles. If you fancy an added challenge, keep these muscles switched on and your shoulders anchored as you slowly spin your fingers to point forward again, holding here for another 5 breaths. You have then definitely earned yourself another "child's pose" (see page 85).

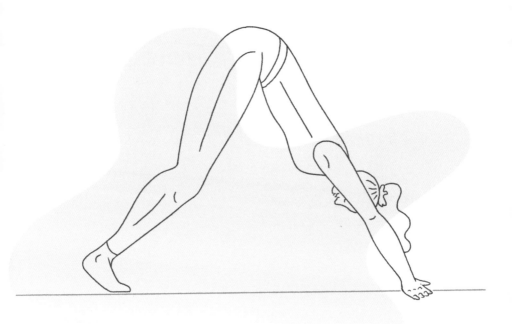

○ Morning routine

○ Micro-moment

○ Daily daylight awe walk

○ Movement inspiration

○ Evening wind down

Day 20.
Micro-moments:
digestion and release

SEATED SPINE TWIST

This one can be done while sitting at your desk, or, if you are feeling stuck, this can be a tonic while on the toilet itself! Place your feet hip-width apart, breathe in and come into your upright posture. As you exhale, keeping the hips square, rotate your torso to the right, take your hands to your outer right thigh and gaze over your right shoulder. Stay in the twist for a few breaths before exhaling back to centre. Breathe in and affirm your tall posture again before exhaling and twisting to the left. Repeat several times to each side, freeing the spine and stimulating the digestive tract in the process.

TUMMY RUB

Encourage both physical and emotional digestion with this self-massage technique. Place your palms by your right hip, firmly slide them above your navel and over to your left hip, down and around to the right hip again. Repeat the circle in this direction only for a minute.

"SPIKY BALL" MASSAGE

Wake up the soles of your feet by rolling a physiotherapy spiky ball underfoot while sitting at your desk. Notice how this helps you reclaim the dexterity of your toes and brings awareness to your feet. This will emphasize your feeling of being grounded when you stand.

○ Morning routine

○ Micro-moment

○ Daily daylight awe walk

○ Movement inspiration

○ Evening wind down

Day 21.
Mindful downtime

Even though we spend huge chunks of our day sitting, we are not well rested. FOMO is real, and the myth that rest is lazy is perpetuated by our "you snooze you lose" culture. Today we take a look at downtime: how you choose to fill it, and how to remind yourself of good posture during time out.

For many people, relaxation has become synonymous with sedentary screen time. I invite you to reflect on how your tech use is affecting your health and to consider whether you need to flex your boundaries – what is the daily duration of your screen time, what are you engaging with and at what time of day? Jot down in your journal any digital health commitments you'd like to make.

Rest as a practice is a bit of a lost art. The message that our worth is equated with our productivity has us feeling a deep sense of guilt when we stop, and we're so switched on that many people find it hard to relax when they finally do give themselves permission. First, we need to understand clearly what rest is and why it's important, and then we'll build a toolkit of how to do it.

Let's clear up some confusion. Rest does not have to be lying down doing nothing. It might be in stillness, or there could be gentle movement. It might be in silence, or you

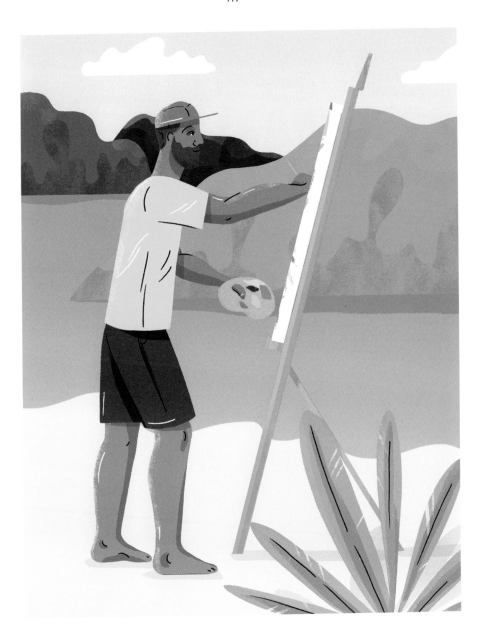

may choose to take in soothing sounds or images. It can be in solitude, or in the company of others. Rest is a feeling of ease, a calm, peaceful state. It is characterized by an absence of overstimulation, effort, striving or pushing. We need restful downtime to heal and restore the mind and body, to recharge, to create space for reflection, for time to digest and process physically and emotionally. The skill of relaxation is also fundamental to our ability to sleep. Far from being lazy, rest can be the most productive choice.

How do we do it? Jot down in your journal a mind map of relaxing activities. Treasured TV, films and gaming count, but keep your posture in mind while you engage in these pursuits and remember to move every 30 minutes. We also need healthy alternatives, and ideally some of these will involve movement. Add to your mind map nourishing tech choices such as audio books, TED talks, podcasts and apps that can guide you in relaxation, stretching, breathing or meditation. Include in your mind map hobbies, creative or expressive outlets such as art, journalling, daydreaming, knitting, reading, vision boarding, doodling, mindful colouring, making music, playing board games, doing jigsaws, sudokus, crosswords, savouring a cup of tea or a good old soak in the tub. For relaxation involving movement, try some "green gazing" in nature's beauty (see page 108), a gentle walk, tenderly massaging in some magnesium body butter, or try the soothing yoga sequence that follows.

Restorative lying-down sequence to destress and stimulate digestion

LYING-DOWN MOUNTAIN BREATHS

Unlike the standing version, which is energizing, this is quietening. Lie down with your legs outstretched, inner ankles and inner knees together, arms by your sides with the palms facing downward. As you breathe in, raise your arms straight up toward the ceiling, then to the floor behind your head, and simultaneously point your toes. (Note: you are not taking your arms out to your sides as with standing "mountain breaths".) As you breathe out, flex your heels and slowly lower your arms back down by your sides. Once this feels comfortable, you could add the coherent breathing ratio of 5 seconds in and 5 seconds out (see page 58). Aim for 5–10 repetitions.

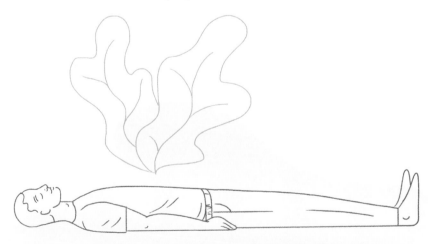

SPINE RELEASE

Hug your knees to your chest and have a little sway side to side. Holding your knees, take them in a circle around your hips, massaging your lower back, 5 times each way.

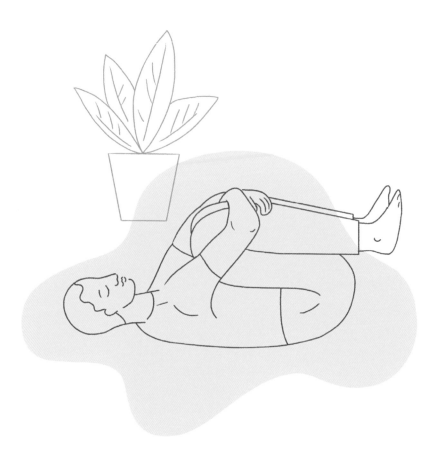

DIGESTIVE PUMPS

Begin with your knees drawn into your chest, take both hands around your right knee, and, as you exhale, slowly stretch your left leg out and down toward the floor, heel flexed, just off the floor. As you breathe in, bring your left leg back in to your chest and bring both hands onto your left knee. As you exhale, slowly stretch your right leg out, heel flexed, hovering off the floor. Inhale and the right leg comes back in. Take your time with this movement. Always start with the right knee in, only one leg moving at a time and one knee staying firmly hugged toward your abdomen throughout, creating a pumping massage for your digestive tract. Aim for 5–10 repetitions on each leg.

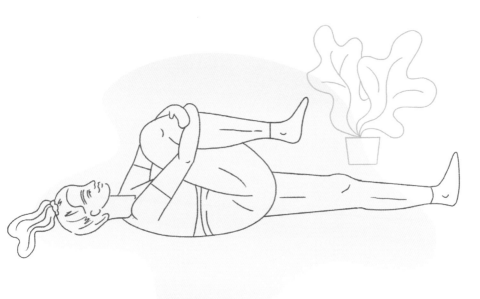

TWIST

Let go with this relaxing twist. Begin with both knees
drawn in to your chest, arms out wide at shoulder height.
Carefully bring your knees over toward your left elbow,
take hold of them with your left hand like an anchor,
and, if comfortable for your neck, look toward your right
up-turned palm. Stay for 5–10 breaths before returning
to the centre and taking your knees over to the right.

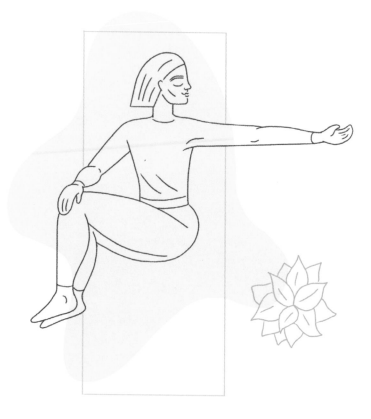

HAPPY BABY

Hug your knees to your chest once more, but this time take your knees wide apart, stretching your inner thighs, and have a little rock here.

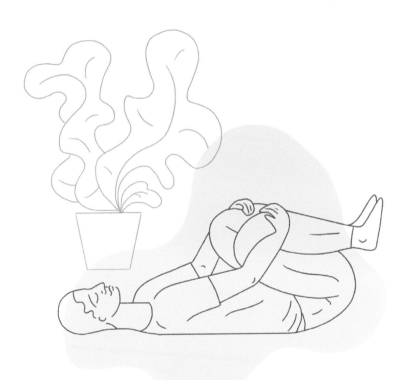

RECLINING BUTTERFLY

Bring your feet flat to the floor and let your knees drop out to your sides, soles of the feet together. If this feels intense for your inner thighs, prop up your knees with cushions. Pop a pillow beneath your head, and, if the temperature calls for it, drape yourself with a soft blanket. We want to maximize comfort here, so consider an eye pillow or warm pack on your abdomen. Lie back and receive fresh energy. If your mind wanders, anchor it on your 5-second breath in and 5-second breath out, or listen to something calming. Hang out here for a few minutes, or as long as you fancy.

○ Morning routine

○ Micro-moment   ○ Movement inspiration

○ Daily daylight awe walk   ○ Evening wind down

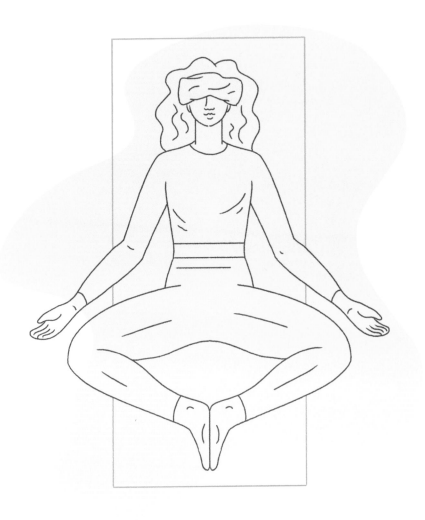

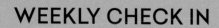

WEEKLY CHECK IN

Congratulations! You are 21 days into the plan. How are you doing with integrating your new habits into your everyday life?

- What kind of benefits are you noticing?
- Take a peek at your entry on day 1 and remember why this is important to you.
- Do your goals need tweaking?

Take stock and reaffirm your commitment to your health and well-being.

Day 22.
Movement breaks:
"wall yoga"

The beauty of this series of poses is that you can work deeply but feel safe and supported by a wall, developing both strength and suppleness. Warm up your body first with some "mountain breaths" from your morning routine and the "tai chi sumo squat" (see pages 56 and 76).

TRIANGLE POSE AGAINST THE WALL

Locate an expanse of wall space that you can lean back into unimpeded. Start facing away from the wall with your feet 5cm (2 inches) away from the base, hands to hips, and lean your buttocks into the wall. Stride your feet one and a half times your shoulder-width apart, turn your right toes to point out and slide your left heel away from you, which will lean your right buttock into the wall. Keep your left leg firmly straight, bend your right knee a little and lean your shoulders evenly into the wall behind you. Without letting your right buttock or shoulders draw away from the wall, slowly slide your right hand to your right shin, hinging deeply at your right hip. Reach your left arm straight up, pressing it into the wall for support, and look down at your right foot.

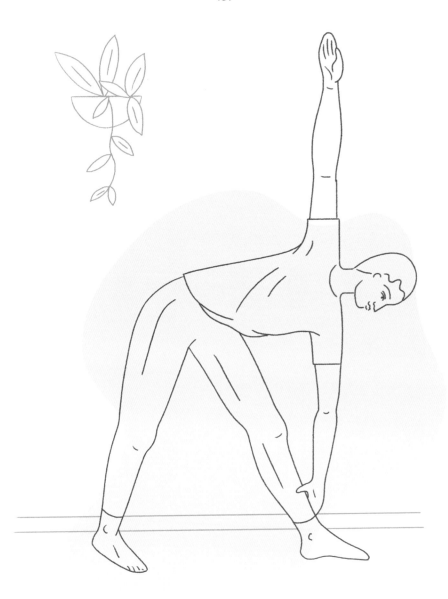

This is a powerful stretch for your right inner thigh and the left-hand side of your chest and you'll feel the muscles behind your left shoulder leap into action, too. Hang out here for 5–10 breaths before slowly rising and taking the pose over to the left.

WIDE LEG FOLD AGAINST THE WALL

Take your feet now to twice shoulder-width apart and turn your toes a fraction inward so the outer edges of your feet are parallel. Bring hands to hips, rest your buttocks into the wall behind you and generously bend your knees. Keeping your knees soft and hips pressed into the wall, slowly drape your torso forward, either touching your fingertips to the floor, your hands to your ankles, or holding onto your elbows. Allow the crown of your head to drop toward the floor, releasing your spine. Take 5–10 breaths here before returning your hands to your hips and slowly rising back up on an inhalation. Notice how much taller you feel after this sequence.

○ Morning routine

○ Micro-moment   ○ Movement inspiration

○ Daily daylight awe walk   ○ Evening wind down

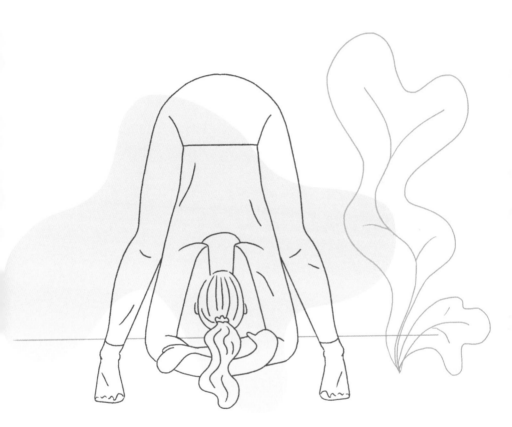

Day 23.
Movement breaks:
posture clinic

DOOR FRAME HANG

Stand in your tall posture in an open doorway with your right shoulder inside the frame. Reach your left arm up and overhead and take a firm grip of the door frame with your left hand, your right arm relaxed by your side. Keeping your body square (so no twisting, arching or rounding), lean your body weight to your left, enjoying a deep stretch on the left-hand side of your torso. Stay here for 5–10 breaths before turning around, changing sides. When you release the intercostal muscles between the ribs, there is more space for each fresh new inhalation, boosting your energy and concentration. Notice how different your breathing and posture feel after this releases the sides of your body.

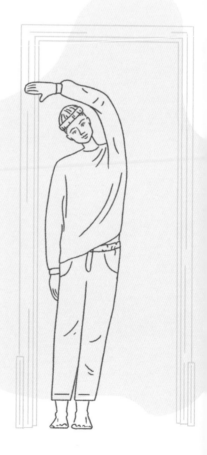

CHEST OPENER

Stand in an open doorway
with your right shoulder
inside the door frame, then
place the length of your right
forearm on the wall within the
door, so that your elbow is at
a right angle and your upper
arm is parallel to the floor.
Take a small step forward
with your right foot and bend
your right knee until you feel a
stretch in the right-hand side
of your chest. Enjoy 5–10 calm
breaths here before turning
around, repeating on your left
side. Feel the impact on your
breathing and the buoyancy
given to your ribcage.

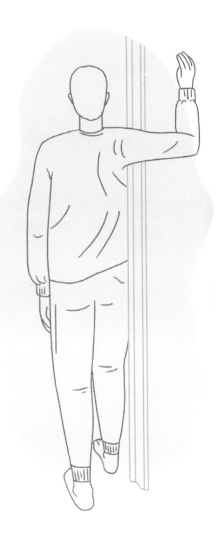

○ Morning routine

○ Micro-moment

○ Daily daylight awe walk

○ Movement inspiration

○ Evening wind down

Day 24.
Micro-moments:
emotional letting go

JAW MASSAGE

Firmly run your fingertips from your outer cheekbones straight down to your lower jaw, letting your mouth open as you do so. Allow this to release all those words you didn't say.

LION BREATH

Inhale slowly through your nose and, as you exhale, stick your tongue out as far as you can with a cathartic roar. Repeat several times, as necessary, allowing pent-up anger, resentment and frustration to leave your body without doing harm.

TEMPORAL PRESS

Create a feeling of being safe and held by cupping your chin in your hands and wrapping your fingertips to your temples. Apply gentle pressure and remember: you can be your own safe place.

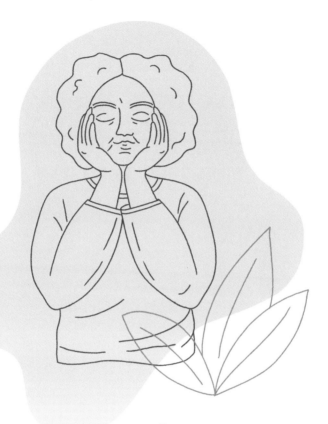

○ Morning routine

○ Micro-moment

○ Daily daylight awe walk

○ Movement inspiration

○ Evening wind down

Day 25.
Movement breaks:
boosting circulation and
mental clarity

WOOD CHOPPER

Stand with your feet one and a half times your shoulder-width apart, toes pointing forward. Start by breathing in and raising your arms upward with your palms touching. As you exhale, bend your knees and bring your hands to touch your outer left knee. Breathe in, and, with vigour, sweep your hands up and across your body on a diagonal line to the right. Exhale while you chop your hands down to the left once more. Repeat 10 times, feeling the strength of your legs and core as you move. Shake out your arms and legs before repeating to the other side.

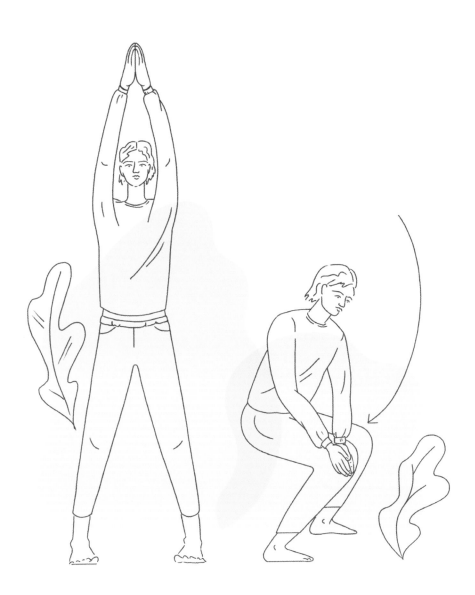

BALANCING CALF RAISE MOUNTAIN

Stand with feet hip-width apart, your gaze forward and your palms flat on the front of your thighs. As you breathe in, raise your arms forward and up overhead, simultaneously raising your heels, keeping your gaze forward. Expect to wobble! As you exhale, slowly lower your heels and your hands back down, ideally both returning to their starting place at the same time. It is easier said than done! Take at least 5 of these, noticing how impossible it is to think about anything else at the same time. The means it's the perfect circuit breaker when unhelpful thoughts arise.

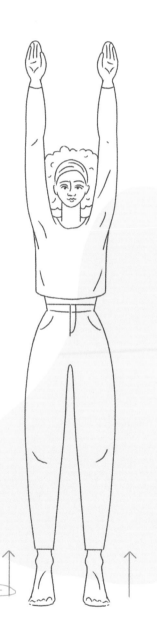

STANDING TWIST

When mind fog descends, get up on your feet and shake it off. With your feet shoulder-width apart, take a dynamic twist, swinging your arms ragdoll-style to the right, looking over your right shoulder and allowing your left heel to lift. Swing your arms over to the left, looking over your left shoulder and allowing your right heel to lift and deepen the twist. Nothing fancy required, just imagine any heaviness flicking from your fingertips. Repeat 5 times on each side, feeling lighter and brighter with each sway.

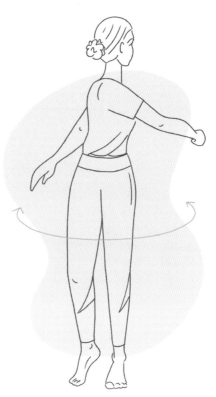

○ Morning routine

○ Micro-moment

○ Daily daylight awe walk

○ Movement inspiration

○ Evening wind down

Day 26.
Movement breaks:
boosting confidence and mood

STANDING MOVEMENT

The best movement to lift
you up is a fluid action with
swinging arms and an upright
spine, such as high-knee
skipping on the spot, or with
travel, if you have space[32].

ARM SLIDES

This will help to strengthen
the muscles that hold you
in a position of power and
poise. Sit tall, feet flat on
the floor and gaze forward
throughout. As you breathe
in, raise your arms up to a "V"
shape with your hands wide
and your palms facing each
other. Stretch up through all
your fingers, especially the

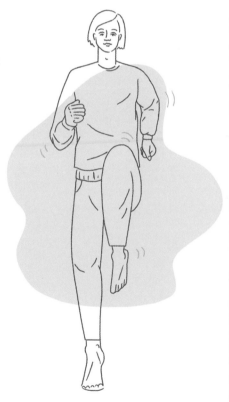

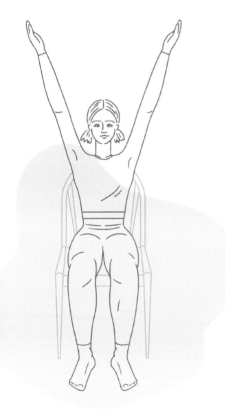

little fingers, but keep the shoulders away from your ears. As you breathe out, slide your elbows downward forming a "W" shape with your arms, broadening your chest, sliding your shoulder blades down your back and keeping the fingertips splayed wide. Repeat 5–10 times, using your *"I am"* intention statement from Day 9 (see page 80) for added effect.

○ Morning routine

○ Micro-moment

○ Daily daylight awe walk

○ Movement inspiration

○ Evening wind down

Day 27.
Movement breaks:
finding balance

STANDING KNEE HUGS

Sense of humour engaged, prepare to wobble! Stand close to a wall, so if you need support, you can reach out and steady yourself. Begin with feet hip-width apart, gazing forward and keeping your spine elongated throughout. As you breathe in, raise your right knee as high as you can and hug it with both hands toward your chest, feeling a stretch in the right-hand side of your lower back. As you exhale, slowly lower your right foot back to the ground. Inhale and raise your left knee high, hugging it to your chest, then release it back down with the exhalation. Keep alternating sides, moving

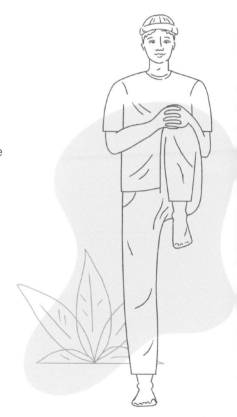

as slowly and with as much control as possible. To maximize the engagement of your legs and core muscles, flex powerfully the heel of the foot you are raising. Feel how this helps you balance, and, as your strength builds, so will your ability to balance in this precarious sequence. Make 5–10 repetitions on each leg, strengthening your buttocks and core and releasing your lower back.

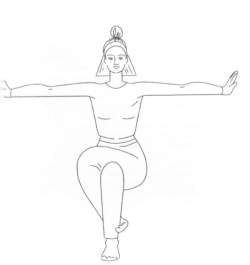

EAGLE LEGS

Get ready to greet your inner thighs! Start in a mini squat with your arms out to your sides, hands held out like a double stop sign. Lift your right knee up and wrap it up and over your left knee so there is no daylight between your thighs. If possible, wrap your right toes behind your left calf. Don't worry if this second wrap isn't accessible. Now sink a little lower into the squat, pressing your thighs deeply toward each other, and, while breathing smoothly, draw your navel toward your spine. Sit with it for 5–10 breaths before shaking out your legs and repeating to the other side. This provides a powerful stretch for your outer thighs while strengthening your core and inner thighs.

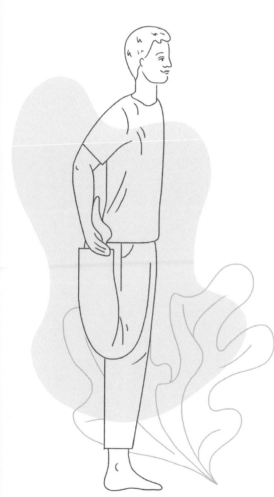

QUAD RELEASE

Stand tall and take your right heel to your right buttock, keeping a little softness in your left knee. Hold onto your right ankle with your right hand, and, if you're up for an extra challenge, see if you can take hold with both hands. Your "embellishment" in this shape is to keep your knees firmly together and point your tailbone down toward the floor, deepening the stretch for the front of your thigh (quadriceps) and hip (hip flexor). If you want to deepen the stretch further, see if you can slide your right knee back behind you a touch. Take 5–10 breaths here before releasing and repeating on the other side.

LET IT ALL GO WITH A WALL FORWARD BEND ADAPTED FROM DAY 22 (SEE PAGE 132)

This time, rather than wide legs, bring your feet to hip-width apart, and, keeping your knees generously bent, hang out here for 5–10 breaths. This is a nice way to close this balance sequence, stretching out your spine and hamstrings and bringing your body back to symmetry.

○ Morning routine

○ Micro-moment

○ Daily daylight awe walk

○ Movement inspiration

○ Evening wind down

Day 28.
Check in and celebrate your accomplishments!

Well done! You have arrived at day 28! Take a look at your notes and recall your baseline (see page 50).

- **What's changed for you? Things may have changed significantly, or maybe you're just getting going.**

Wherever you've ended up, it's ok. If you haven't made as much headway as you would've liked, that's ok, too! Change is challenging for us human beings, so go gently and remember self-compassion is key (see page 88). You can take your time!

Reward not only progress but effort. How can you give yourself a pat on the back that supports your progress?

To sustain the benefits you're seeing, you need to keep going, so jot down what your next steps might be. Is there a new goal you'd like to work towards, or a different aspect of your well-being that you're interested to develop?

You could even go back through this 28-day plan in entirety, working on any suggestions you skipped, or any that didn't resonate or stick as a habit the first time around. Try again: it might feel different this time, especially as your mindfulness muscles and fitness improve. Keep mixing it up, cherry-picking the days that speak to you in the moment, adding to your well-being toolkits. Identify the next wave of change, or, if you've found your groove, just keep it up! I'm cheering you on!

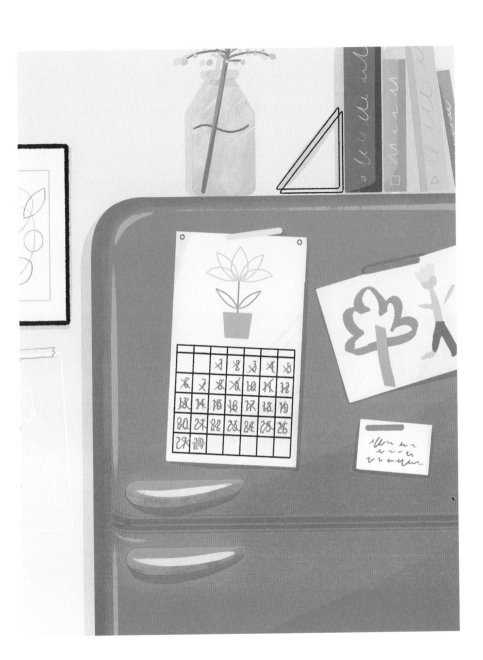

References

[1] American Heart Association, 'The Price of Inactivity', 2015
atgprod.heart.org/HEARTORG/HealthyLiving/PhysicalActivity/FitnessBasics/
The-Price-of-Inactivity_UCM_307974_Article.jsp

[2] British Heart Foundation, Physical Inactivity and Sedentary Behaviour Report, 2017
www.bhf.org.uk

[3] Insana, Ron, 'Getting Inspiration from the Greatest Generation's Economic Hardship
and Shared Sacrifice', CNBC, 2020
cnbc.com/2020/03/29/op-ed-getting-inspiration-from-the-greatest-generations-eco-
nomic-hardship-and-shared-sacrifice.html

[4] Tison, Geoffrey H; Avram, Robert; Kuhar, Peter, 'Worldwide Effect of COVID-19 on
Physical Activity: A Descriptive Study', *Annals of Internal Medicine*, 2020
acpjournals.org/doi/10.7326/M20-2665

[5] Morris, J N; Crawford, M D, 'Coronary Heart-disease and Physical Activity of Work;
Evidence of a National Necropsy Survey', National Library of Medicine, 1958
pubmed.ncbi.nlm.nih.gov/13110049

[6] Morris, J N; Heady, J A; Raffle, P A B; Roberts, C G; Parks, J W, 'Coronary Heart-disease
and Physical Activity of Work', *The Lancet*, 1953
thelancet.com/journals/lancet/article/PIIS0140-6736(53)91495-0/fulltext

[7] Taylor, Henry Longstreet; Klepetar, Ernest; Keys, Ancel; Parlin, Willis; Blackburn, Henry;
Puchner, Thomas, 'Death Rates Among Physically Active and Sedentary Employees of
the Railroad Industry', *American Journal of Public Health*, 1962
ncbi.nlm.nih.gov/pmc/articles/PMC1523019

[8] Gilchrist, Susan C; Howard, Virginia J; Akinyemiju, Tomi; et al, 'Association of Sedentary Behaviour with Cancer Mortality in Middle-aged and Older US Adults', JAMA
Health Forum, 2020
jamanetwork.com/journals/jamaoncology/article-abstract/2767093

[9] Siddarth, Prabha; Burggren, Alison C; Eyre, Harris A; Small, Gary W; Merrill, David A,
'Sedentary Behaviour Associated with Reduced Medial Temporal Lobe Thickness in
Middle-aged and Older Adults', PLOS ONE, 2018
journals.plos.org/plosone/article?id=10.1371/journal.pone.0195549

[10] Patterson, Richard; McNamara, Eoin; Tainio, Marko; Hérick de Sá, Thiago; Smith, Andrea D; Sharp, Stephen J; Edwards, Phil; Woodcock, James; Brage, Søren; Wijndaele, Katrien, 'Sedentary Behaviour and Risk of All-cause, Cardiovascular and Cancer Mortality, and Incident Type 2 Diabetes: a Systematic Review and Dose Response Meta-analysis', *European Journal of Epidemiology*, 2018
link.springer.com/article/10.1007/s10654-018-0380-1

[11] Park, Jung Ha; Moon, Ji Hyun; Kim, Hyeon Ju; Kong, Mi Hee; Oh, Yun Hwan, 'Sedentary Lifestyle: Overview of Updated Evidence of Potential Health Risks', *Korean Journal of Family Medicine*, 2020
pubmed.ncbi.nlm.nih.gov/33242381

[12] Hamilton, Marc T; Healy, Genevieve N; Dunstan, David W; Zderic, Theodore W; Owen, Neville, 'Too Little Exercise and Too Much Sitting: Inactivity Physiology and the Need for New Recommendations on Sedentary Behaviour', *Curr Cardiovascular Risk Report*, 2008
ncbi.nlm.nih.gov/pmc/articles/PMC3419586

[13] Ekelund, Ulf; Steene-Johannessen, Jostein; Brown, Wendy J; Fagerland, Morten W; Owen, Neville; Powell, Kenneth E; et al, 'Does Physical Activity Attenuate, or Even Eliminate, the Detrimental Association of Sitting Time with Mortality? A Harmonised Meta-analysis of Data from More Than 1 Million Men and Women', *The Lancet*, 2016
thelancet.com/pdfs/journals/lancet/PIIS0140-6736(16)30370-1.pdf

[14] Healy, Genevieve N; Dunstan, David W; Salmon, Jo; Cerin, Esther; Shaw, Jonathan E; Zimmet, Paul Z; Owen, Neville, 'Breaks in Sedentary Time: Beneficial Associations with Metabolic Risk', *Diabetes Care*, 1008
pubmed.ncbi.nlm.nih.gov/18252901

[15] Lee, I-Min; Shiroma, Eric J; Lobelo, Felipe; Puska, Pekka; Blair, Steven N; Katzmarzyk, Peter T, 'Effect of Physical Inactivity on Major Non-communicable Diseases Worldwide: an Analysis of Burden of Disease and Life Expectancy', *The Lancet*, 2012
thelancet.com/journals/lancet/article/PIIS0140-6736(12)61031-9/fulltext

[16] Reynolds, Gretchen, 'Sitting All Day May Increase Your Risk of Dying from Cancer', *The New York Times*, 2020
https://www.nytimes.com/2020/06/24/well/move/sitting-sedentary-exercise-cancer-risk.html

[17] Mandsager, Kyle; Harb, Serge; Cremer, Paul; et al, 'Association of Cardiorespiratory Fitness with Long-term Mortality Among Adults Undergoing Exercise Treadmill Testing', JAMA Network, 2018
jamanetwork.com/journals/jamanetworkopen/fullarticle/2707428

[18] Heron, Leonie; O'Neill, Ciaran; McAneney, Helen; Kee, Frank; Tully, Mark A, 'Direct Healthcare Costs of Sedentary Behaviour in the UK', *BMJ Journals*, 2019 jech.bmj.com/content/73/7/625.info

[19] Raichlen, David A; Pontzer, Herman; Zderic, Theodore W; Harris, Jacob A; Mabulla, Audax Z P; Hamilton, Marc T; Wood, Brian M, 'Sitting, Squatting, and the Evolutionary Biology of Human Inactivity', PNAS, 2020 pnas.org/content/117/13/7115

[20] Ekeland, Ulf; Tarp, Jakob; Fagerland, Morten W; Steele-Johannessen, Jostein; Hansen, Bjørge H; Jefferis, Barbara J; Whincup, Peter H; Diaz, Keith M; Hooker, Steven; Howard, Virginia J; Chernofsky, Ariel; Larson, Martin G; Spartano, Nicole; Vasan, Ramachandran S; Dohrn, Ing-Mari; Hagströmer, Maria; Edwardson, Charlotte; Yates, Thomas; Shiroma, Eric; Dempsey, Paddy; Wijndaele, Katrien; Anderssen, Sigmund A; Lee, I-Min, 'Joint Associations of Accelerometer-measured Physical Activity and Sedentary Time with All-cause Mortality: a Harmonised Meta-analysis in More Than 44,000 Middle-aged and Older Individuals', *British Journal of Sports Medicine*, 2020 bjsm.bmj.com/content/54/24/1499

[21] Wolfe, Anthony S; Burton, Heath M; Vardarli, Emre; Coyle, Edward F, 'Hourly 4-s Sprints Prevent Impairment of Postprandial Fat Metabolism from Inactivity', *Medicine & Science in Sports & Exercise*, 2020 journals.lww.com/acsm-msse/Citation/2020/10000/Hourly_4_s_Sprints_Prevent_Impairment_of.23.aspx

[22] O'Donovan, Gary; Lee, I-Min; Hamer, Mark; et al, 'Association of "Weekend Warrior" and Other Leisure Time Physical Activity Patterns with Risks for All-cause, Cardiovascular Disease, and Cancer Mortality', JAMA Network, 2017 jamanetwork.com/journals/jamainternalmedicine/article-abstract/2596007

[23] Endrighi, Romano; Steptoe, Andrew; Hamer, Mark, 'The Effect of Experimentally Induced Sedentariness on Mood and Psychobiological Responses to Mental Stress', *British Journal of Psychiatry*, 2016 pubmed.ncbi.nlm.nih.gov/26294364

[24] Peper, Erik, 'Posture Affects Memory Recall and Mood', *The Peper Pespective*, 2017 peperperspective.com/2017/11/25/posture-affects-memory-recall-and-mood

[25] Peper, Erik, '"Don't slouch!" Improve Health with Posture Feedback', *The Peper Perspective*, 2019 peperperspective.com/2019/07/01/dont-slouch-improves-health-with-posture-feedback

[26] Schuch, Felipe B; Vancampfort, Davy; Firth, Joseph; Rosenbaum, Simon; Ward, Philip B; Silva, Edson S; Hallgren, Mats; Ponce de Leon, Antonio; Dunn, Andrea L; Deslandes, Andrea C; Fleck, Marcelo P; Carvalho, Andre F; Stubbs, Brendon, 'Physical Activity and Incident Depression: a Meta-analysis of Prospective Cohort Studies', *The American Journal of Psychiatry*, 2018
ajp.psychiatryonline.org/doi/10.1176/appi.ajp.2018.17111194

[27] Knapton, Sarah, 'Exercising for 20 Minutes a Day Cuts Risk of Developing Depression by One-third', *The Daily Telegraph*, 2018
telegraph.co.uk/science/2018/04/24/exercising-20-minutes-a-day-cuts-risk-developing-depression

[28] Russo, Marc A; Santarella, Danielle M; O'Rourke, Dean, 'The Physiological Effects of Slow Breathing in the Healthy Human', *Breathe*, 2017
ncbi.nlm.nih.gov/pmc/articles/PMC5709795

[29] Sturm, V E; Datta, S; Roy, A R K; Sible, I J; Kosik, E L; Veziris, C R; Chow, T E; Morris, N A; Neuhaus, J; Kramer, J H; Miller, B L; Holley, S R; Keltner, D, 'Big Smile, Small Self: Awe Walks Promote Prosocial Positive Emotions in Older Adults', American Psychological Association, 2020
psycnet.apa.org/doiLanding?doi=10.1037%2Femo0000876

[30] Adams, Claire E; Leary, Mark R, 'Promoting Self-compassionate Attitudes Toward Eating Among Restrictive and Guilty Eaters', *Journal of Social and Clinical Psychology*, 2007
self-compassion.org/wp-content/uploads/publications/AdamsLearyeating_attitudes.pdf

[31] Moser, Jason S; Dougherty, Adrienne; Mattson, Whitney I; Katz, Benjamin; Moran, Tim P; Guevarra, Darwin; Shablack, Holly; Ayduk, Ozlem; Jonides, John; Berman, Marc G; Kross, Ethan, 'Third-person Self-talk Facilitates Emotion Regulation without Engaging Cognitive Control: Converging Evidence from ERP and fMRI', *Nature Briefing*, 2017
nature.com/articles/s41598-017-04047-3

[32] Peper, Erik; Lin, I-Mei; Harvey, Richard; Perez, Jacob, 'How Posture Affects Memory Recall and Mood', *Biofeedback*, 2017
biofeedbackhealth.files.wordpress.com/2017/11/0-article-biof-45-02-36-41.pdf

Index

Acknowledgements

Deepest thanks to Dave, Charlotte and Ted for helping me carve the time, space and energy to write this book despite the squeeze of lockdown.

I am indebted to Kate Adams, my Consultant Publisher for her forward thinking and championing of this timely book.

As ever, a deep bow of gratitude to my agent Jane Graham Maw, for her encouragement and impeccable advocacy.

This book is very much a collective achievement and my heartfelt appreciation goes to Senior Editor Pauline Bache, Art Director Yasia Williams, illustrator Abi Read and PR maven Megan Brown. This book has been such a joy to create and I am so thankful to you all for helping me bring it to life in such a colourful, accessible way.

Thanks to all my readers, your kind words genuinely spur me on, and to all the kindred spirits who gather with me for our weekly Instagram #MondayMicroMoment live sessions, thank you for being part of the real caring community there. We lift each other up.

I so look forward to seeing the upward spiral of positivity this little book will set into motion! Thank YOU for sharing the journey with me.